Frank Arjava Petter · Tadao Yamaguchi · Chujiro Hayashi

The Hayashi Reiki Manual

Traditional Japanese Healing Techniques
from the Founder of the Western Reiki System

LOTUS PRESS
SHANGRI-LA

Important Note:
The information presented in this book has been carefully researched and passed on according to our best knowledge and conscience. However, the author and publisher assume no liability whatsoever for damages of any kind that occur directly from the application or use of the statements in this book. This information is meant as further education for interested parties.
The methods of healing and exercises listed in this book are no substitute for consulting a physician or naturopath. They are meant to support the healing process as an additional treatment. The laws of the USA permit the practice of medicine only by registered physicians and healing practitioners who have been trained in accordance with the law.

First English Reprint 2018
First English Edition 2003
© by Lotus Press
Box 325, Twin Lakes, WI 53181, USA
website: www.lotuspress.com
email: lotuspress@lotuspress.com
The Shangri-La Series is published in cooperation
with Schneelöwe Verlagsberatung, Federal Republic of Germany
© 2002 by Windpferd Verlagsgesellschaft mbH, Aitrang, Germany All
rights reserved
Cover design by Kuhn Graphik, Digitales Design, Zurich, Switzerland
by using a photo of Shouya P. T. Grigg
Photos on pages 8, 19, and 28 © Tadao Yamaguchi
Photos of the Reiki techniques by Shouya P. T. Grigg
Editing by Neehar Douglass

ISBN 978-0-9149-5575-7
Library of Congress Control Number 2003103528

Dedication

Dedicated to the sacred memory of
Chujiro and Chie Hayashi.

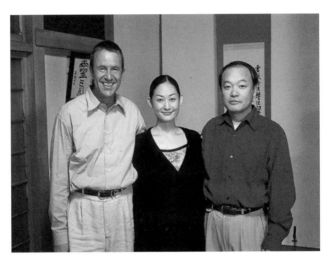

Frank Arjava Petter, Nanako Itoh, Tadao Yamaguchi

We would like to thank:

Chiyoko Yamaguchi and her family for the wealth of knowledge they have shared with us all.

Shouya P.T. Grigg for taking the wonderful photos of the healing techniques.

Our editor Neehar Douglass for his professional support.

Our supermodel Nanako Itoh for her dedicated work.

Mr. Hiroshi Tamura for the original Reiki certificates signed by Dr. Hayashi and Dr. Hayashi's stamp on pages 6 and 36.

Mitsue Yamada for the background information about Dr. Hayashi.

Ikuko Hirota and Amanda Jayne for translating chapters 1 to 3 from Japanese into English.

Chetna M. Kobayashi for her assistance in translating the Ryoho Shishin in chapter 5.

Alongside this Arjava thanks Bhakti for her devotion.

And of course the Windpferd team who has helped this book become reality.

Table of Contents

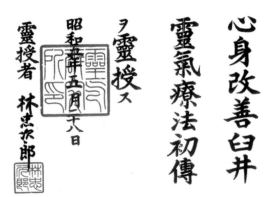

心身改善臼井靈氣療法初傳

寺坂とよ

ヲ靈授ス

昭和五年五月十八日

靈授者　林忠次郎

Original Reiki certificate signed by Dr. Chujiro Hayashi

6

The Prophecy

There is a prophecy on the tombstone of Mikao Usui, the founder of Reiki, that the practice of Reiki will spread all over the world, healing the people as well as Planet Earth herself.

This epitaph to a beloved teacher was written in 1927 by Juzaburo Ushida the second chairperson of the Usui Reiki Ryoho Gakkai, Dr. Usui's Reiki organization. Little did he know the explosive effect Reiki would have on Mother Earth and all of her children.

Today Reiki is practiced on all continents by people of all creeds and races, social status and of all religions. This fact is due to the dedicated effort of one man and one man alone, Dr Chujiro Hayashi.

In the mid-nineteen thirties after he had broken away from the Usui Reiki Ryoho Gakkai Dr Hayashi teamed up with Hawayo Takata in Hawaii and with her help brought Reiki to the USA. This was the great step. The rest of the story is history... Reiki spread from Hawaii to America and from there to Europe, to Australia, to Asia and Africa.

In the winter of 1999 I learned of an old lady who had been a direct disciple of Chujiro Hayashi. This lady was said to be teaching in Kyoto, my favorite city in Japan. Her name, I heard, was Mrs. Yamaguchi. For seven years I had been looking for the possibility of training with someone who had learned the traditional form of Reiki in Japan.

Before I called the Yamaguchis I was not really full of hope. Would they even talk to me once they discovered that I was a foreigner? However I was determined to find out.

Already on the telephone Tadao Yamaguchi was very open, friendly and polite. He didn't mind at all that I was foreign or that I had been teaching Reiki for seven years. Actually he was thrilled that I wanted to train with him and his mother.

Several months later, in the summer of 2000, I spent five days in Kyoto with Mrs. Chiyoko Yamaguchi and her son Tadao. I was to learn Reiki One and Reiki Two just as Dr. Hayashi had taught them sixty years before. What an exciting prospect being able to immerse myself in the original Reiki as taught by Dr Hayashi himself!

I wondered about the attunements, the symbols, the hand positions and so on. But what I was looking forward to most was to see and feel how someone

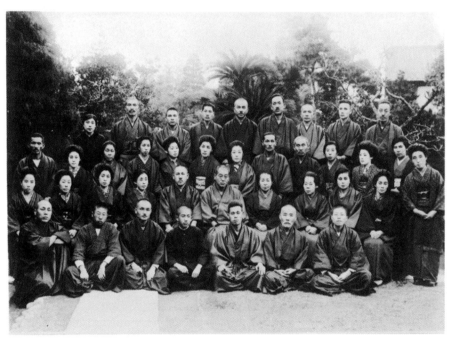

**Dr. Mikao Usui—sixth from left in second row and
Dr. Chujiro Hayashi—forth from right in top row**

who had practiced Reiki her whole life would BE. I was disappointed with the way many Western Reiki teachers live their lives and how they do not live what they teach.

Meeting One of Dr. Hayashi's Students

Meeting Mrs. Yamaguchi and her family heralded a new era in Reiki for me. As I left the Yamaguchi home in Kyoto after this first initiation I told Mrs. Yamaguchi what an immense pleasure it had been for me to finally meet an honorable Reiki Master'. In the Western World we are still in the adolescent stage of Reiki. What we call "tradition" is at the most twenty-five years old. In the presence of Mrs. Yamaguchi I felt the spirit of Reiki being transmitted with extreme clarity. I found Reiki in every smile, in every reassuring word this humble lady uttered, in every little healing hint she gave. In the way she moves, in the way she talks and lives in each moment of her life.

A year later I visited the Yamaguchi's again. During this step in my training our friendship and the mutual trust that was growing in our hearts further matured. Tadao Yamaguchi and I even decided we would write a book together.

In the summer of 2002 my dream came true and I began The Reiki Master Training under the Yamaguchis. This was the completion of one full cycle in my life. I left Japan and am living now in Germany, returning to my roots.

Those of you who are familiar with my other Reiki books know that I have focused mostly on Dr. Usui and the way he taught, somewhat neglecting Dr. Hayashi. This was not intentional but from a lack of knowledge. I am very happy that Tadao Yamaguchi has shone light onto this missing piece in the Reiki puzzle.

In this book we offer you the Hayashi Reiki Ryoho Shishin (Reiki treatment plan) in a fresh translation, illustrated with photographs and graphics to make it easy for you to use.

We describe the most important techniques without which this approach to Reiki cannot be understood. You will also find a number of photographs and other material never before published, as well as the Yamaguchi family story in the light of Reiki.

We hope that the information in this book and the love flowing from between the lines will inspire you dear reader and will bring to you what it has given us. May your hands and the people they touch benefit from the journey you are about to embark upon.

Historical Part

Chapter 1

Chujiro Hayashi's Life*

Hayashi's life followed a quite individual path on the one hand and, on the other, he was well connected into the social fabric of his time. To give an idea of this, a sketch showing some of the steps in his life follows:

Mr. Chujiro Hayashi was born in Tokyo on September 15th 1880. He graduated from the 30th class at the Japan Naval Academy in 1902, serving in the Port Patrolling Division during the Russo-Japanese War from February 4th of that year until a peace treaty concluded that war on September 5th 1906.

In 1918 he was appointed Director of Ominato Port Defence Station where Kanichi Taketomi (later to become the 3rd chairman of Usui Ryoho Gakkai) was the Chief of Staff.**

Ominato was a port located at the foot of Mt Osore on the Shimokita Peninsula in Aomori in the North of Japan. At that time defense ports were second in importance only to Naval Base ports.

Mr. Hayashi was married with two children. His wife Chie was born in 1887 and they married after she graduated from Shizuoka Women's High School. Their first child Tadayoshi, born in 1903 went on to major in economics at Keio University. Kiyoe their second child, born 7 years later studied at the same school as her mother.

In 1935 they lived at 28 Higashi-shinano-cho, Yotsuya, Tokyo (now known as 27 Shinano-cho, Shinjuku ward, Tokyo). This was the year that Chiyoko Yamaguchi first met Mr. Hayashi. It was at this address that he ran his considerable Reiki clinic. The clinic consisted of 10 tables on which patients each received treatment via 2 practitioners.

He actively promoted Reiki throughout Japan, founding Hayashi Reiki Kenkyu-kai and holding seminars teaching Reiki to a great number of people.

Chujiro Hayashi ended his life at his villa in Atami, a hot spring resort near Mt Fuji, on May 11th 1940.

---

* Source: "Taishu-Jinjiroku" (general biographical dictionary) published in 1940.

** Juzaburo Ushida the second chairman of Usui Ryoho Gakkai (from 1926 until 1935) was a captain in the Japanese navy. After Kanichi Taketomi (3rd chairman starting in 1935), Hoichi Wanami the fifth chairman (until 1975) was also in the navy as a submarine commanding officer.
  —These data are from the official staff lists of the Japanese navy.

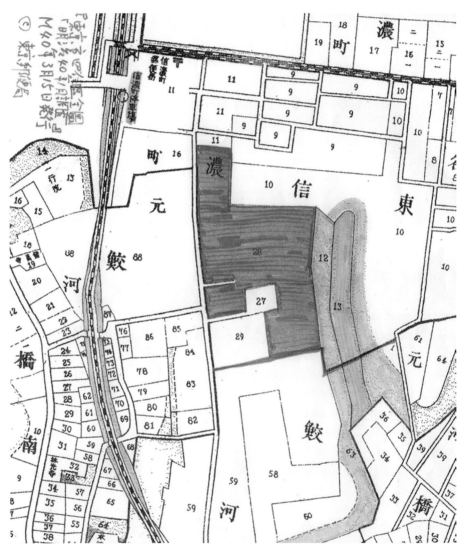

The old map of Tokyo also shows Dr. Chujiro Hayasi's Reiki clinic (in the middle)

Chapter 2

The Yamaguchi Family Story in Connection to Reiki

My Family's First Encounter with Reiki

Mr. Wasaburo Sugano, my mother's uncle, first brought Reiki into my family. He was a hardworking man from Ishikawa in the North of Japan who moved to Osaka to start his career. There he worked his way up to become executive director of his company.

Sugano Sensei's* initial interest in Reiki was spurred by the sad deaths of both of his children. His first child died soon after birth and his second at the age of 15 from tuberculosis, which in those days was considered to be incurable.

Success, with all the money power and status that it brings, could not save his children for him. Conventional medicine offered nothing. He was completely helpless. Hearing about Reiki Ryoho (treatment) by chance, these bitter, painful experiences prompted his initial interest and led him to his first Reiki seminar.

So it was that Wasaburo Sugano Sensei first learned Reiki Ryoho directly from Chujiro Hayashi Sensei in Sakai, Osaka, in 1928.

As Sugano Sensei became proficient in the practice of Reiki (he had progressed from the 6th degree *Shoden* to *Okuden***) he actively promoted the treatments amongst his extended family and his co-workers in Osaka. Many were invited to Osaka from his home-town of Daishoji in Ishikawa district.

The exact nature of the degree system at that time is unclear, however it is known that seminars for studies up to the 3rd degree were held each month. One of the participants who traveled from Ishikawa to Osaka for the 5 days seminar to Shoden level was Katsue Yamaguchi, my mother's elder sister. She

---

* Sensei is a Japanese term of respect for a teacher.

** The traditional Japanese Reiki System is divided onto the following degrees: *Shoden*, the sixth degree is the lowest and represents the First Reiki degree of the Western Reiki System. It is divided into four parts. The next degree is *Okuden* which represents Western Reiki Second Degree. This degree is divided into two parts, Okuden Zenki and Okuden Koki. The next degree, *Shinpiden* is reached by only very few. It is again divided into two parts: Shihan-Kaku (assistant teacher and Shihan (teacher).

fondly remembers these seminars of about 3 hours each day, followed by a practical session where they could give actual treatments and apply what they had learned. However, her treasured memories come not only from her experiences of Reiki but also because among her fellow participants there were several famous Kabuki* actors.

First Reiki Seminar in Daishoji

In Daishoji, district Ishikawa, Reiki treatments were actively given by those who had mastered the practice in Osaka. More and more people were healed and consequently a growing number of people became interested in learning it for themselves. At that time however, travel to Osaka was not easy for them. Few could afford to spend 5 days in a row let alone 50 yen for the tuition (which today is the equivalent of 600,000 yen or US$ 5,500!). A newly graduated teacher was earning 30 yen per month, so the tuition fees were extremely expensive.

These people, hearing that Hayashi Sensei traveled frequently from Tokyo to Osaka as well as to other parts of Japan, invited him to Ishikawa to conduct seminars.

When Wasaburo Sugano Sensei, who had become a great contributor to the expansion of Reiki, put this request to him he happily agreed. He would come if there were more than 10 participants.

These seminars commenced in 1935 and he went regularly to Ishikawa (later known as the Daishoji branch) twice a year in Spring and Autumn.

Hayashi Sensei conducted intensive seminars all over Japan. In 1935 some students achieved *Shihan-kaku* (the assistant teacher degree) and were able to hold *Reiju-Kai* (attunement sessions) when Hayashi Sensei was unavailable. He permitted his students to organize branches in other parts of Japan than Tokyo but, while a number of these branches certainly existed, none, other than the ones in Osaka and Daishoji have been confirmed.

The Daishoji branch was well established by the time my mother Chiyoko Yamaguchi started to learn Reiki in 1938. She was first attuned by Hayashi Sensei himself and admitted to a 5 days seminar where she mingled with students who had already received the *Shihan* (teacher) degree.

---

* Kabuki is traditional Japanese theatre and any Japanese person from her generation would have recognized these actors.

Okuden—The Second Reiki Degree

The first seminar and attunement sessions were held in Daishoji in 1935. Katsue, Chiyoko Yamaguchi's elder sister, participated in these and reached *Okuden*. Hayashi Sensei held Reiki seminars in Tokyo and Osaka every month where students studied through 6th, 5th, 4th, and 3rd degrees leading to *Shoden*. After a number of practise sessions a student developed the ability to feel *Byosen*, problematic areas, and was allowed to proceed to *Okuden* level. This usually took at least 3 months and for some people 6 months to a year, although under the founder of Reiki, Mikao Usui Sensei, achieving *Okuden* level was even more arduous.

Okuden level seminars were usually divided into 2 separate sessions *(Okuden-Zenki* and *Okuden Koki)* but an intensive 5 days course complete was offered for those who traveled long distances.

Chiyoko Yamaguchi's Reiki Path

Chiyoko wanted to learn Reiki from her earliest childhood. It seemed to be the most natural thing for her to do. She grew up strong and health-conscious thanks largely to the use of Reiki within her family. The common home remedy for headaches, stomach aches, colds and fevers was Reiki given by her family members and it always worked. She never had to see any doctors or take any medication. She was often given Reiki by her uncle, aunt and sister.

The more you receive Reiki the more receptive your body becomes, so this experience had laid the ground well when she herself came to learn. Chiyoko observed her sister giving lots of help to their neighbors, effecting recovery from various illnesses via her Reiki. She became more and more convinced of the greatness of Reiki as she saw people coming to thank her sister. She desperately wanted to learn it and as soon as possible.

Her uncle Mr. Sugano had made her wait until she graduated from high school, so she counted down the days impatiently. Finally the great moment arrived.

Chiyoko's First Reiki Attunement

Accompanied by her elder sister Katsue she left the house in the brand new kimono her uncle had brought for the occasion. She was extremely excited but at the same time very nervous. They headed to the house of a member of the Daishoji Reiki branch and found that others, who were much older than Chiyoko, were already there. The atmosphere was quite formal and while her sister who was already a regular member at this branch felt perfectly comfortable, Chiyoko was completely overwhelmed. Her happy mood soon evaporated.

The coordinators greeted the participants with an explanation of the appropriate manner in which to receive *Reiju* (attunement). This, is how my mother was instructed to receive the attunement:

Firstly the room was darkened and they were told to sit in the *Seiza* posture (formal Japanese sitting style on one's knees) with their eyes closed, sitting up straight and taking care no pressure was put on the lower *Tanden* (a spot 3 cm lower than the naval).

Then they put their palms together *(Gassho*—the prayer position) whilst being given *Reiju* which was performed by the placing of a hand on their head from behind. Those giving the attunements touched the participants signaling them as the attunement began to put their hands into the *Gassho* position.

Next they gave another attunement from in front, placing hands around each person's hands in *Gassho*. She waited quietly until all the participants had received this attunement. They were not to stand up or talk. Chiyoko was really nervous but she felt a little more at ease when she found that her aunt was one of the coordinators. She doesn't remember exactly how many participants were there but remembers that there were 3 rows of 5 or 6 *Zabutons* (Japanese cushions for sitting on the floor) and the participants took care to sit on these in an orderly fashion.

After the briefing sessions Hayashi Sensei entered the room dressed in *Haori* and *Hakama* (Japanese formal kimono). Chiyoko was in awe at his dignified appearance and impressive bearing. A tall man he appeared to have light shining all around him. Seeing him Chiyoko was convinced that she was seeing a real halo for the first time.

With Hayashi Sensei leading, *Go-kai-no-sho* (the five Reiki principles written on the scroll that was hung in the room where the attunements took place) were recited. Hayashi Sensei prompted the proceedings by quoting the first line of the pledge *kyo dake wa* (Just for today), then the participants followed by repeating this and the other lines 3 times in unison:

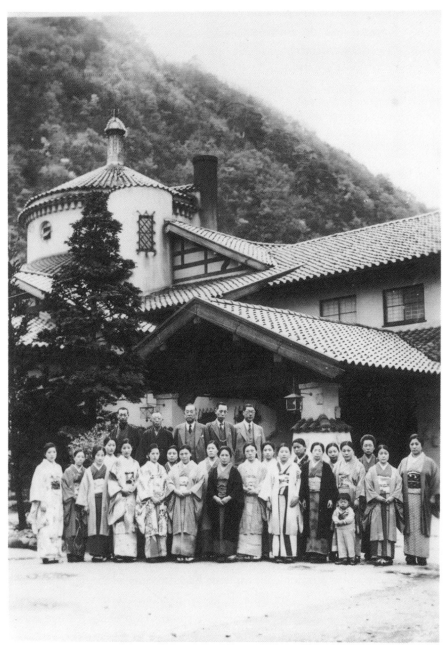

Dr. Chujiro Hayashi—standing in the middle—with students in front of a sanatorium. You can also see Chiyoko Yamaguchi—fifth from right, in the second row

kyo dake wa (Just for today)
ikaru-na (do not get angry)
shinpaisuna (do not worry)
kansha shite (be thankful)
gyo hageme (work hard)
hito-ni shinsetsu-ni (be kind to others)

The light was turned off and the storm shutters closed. The room was so dark that she couldn't read the lines on the scroll.

Then *Reiju* finally began. It was performed by Hayashi Sensei himself followed by the others who held *Shihan* degrees. There were possibly 3 *Shihans*, but she was not sure of the exact number. It was done in such a dark room. Each *Reiju* lasted about 5 minutes and Hayashi Sensei chanted poems written by the Meiji Emperor* throughout the attunement.

After the *Reiju* all the participants came together to form a *Reiki Mawashi* (sitting in a circle, each person laying their hands on the person sitting in front in order to feel the Reiki circulating). Sometimes Hayashi Sensei himself joined the circle and at other times he sat in the center directing the participants.

Hayashi Sensei then went on to explain the theory behind Reiki, using a blackboard to illustrate his points. His lectures were comprehensive but easy to understand for such a young girl at that time.

The Reiki Lectures

The lectures concerned the responsibilities of each person who as a human being has a duty toward all things in the universe. Initially, on this planet, a "divine being" created a "perfect" world for responsible human beings. With the development of civilization we are living more and more comfortably and many of us no longer have to worry about food, clothing or shelter.

However it is clear that we now have more unsolvable problems than ever before. As a result psychological problems have become more serious and diseases have become more complicated. There are many terminal illnesses that conventional medicine cannot treat despite the developments in medical science. Furthermore, our problems are now affecting other living things.

---

* Lübeck/Petter/Rand: *The Spirit of Reiki*, Lotus Press, Twin Lakes, WI, 2001, page 284ff.

Human beings possess their own natural cleansing process or healing power. This enables them to cure themselves of their illnesses, these illnesses in themselves not being harmful. For example when we have a cold we develop a fever. The heat from the fever kills the germs and then removes the toxins from our bodies via our natural waste systems hence it is considered a "natural cleansing process".

However, at some point in time people started to believe that only doctors could cure their illnesses. Today we even mistakenly believe that we have completely recovered from an illness when in fact the pain has only been eased by some palliative. It is far more important to be rid of the underlying problems

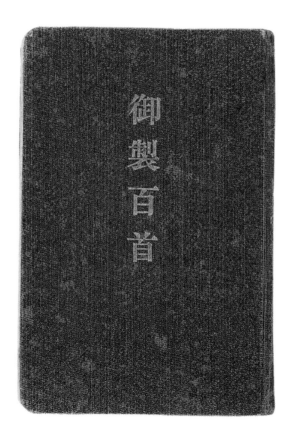

A book containing the Meiji Emperor's poems which Dr. Mikao Usui and also Dr. Chujiro Hayashi recommended to their students

using the body's natural healing powers. However in this modern world most people's natural healing powers are unable to function effectively.

Reiki healers receive cosmic energy (from the sun and the universe beyond). Energy which is amplified and passed to patients via the laying on of hands.

Put simply, Reiki awakens the natural healing powers we all possess but which lie dormant, untapped.

The Muddy Stream ...

Hayashi Sensei often used the image of a "muddy stream" when explaining the natural cleansing process.

When you look at the surface of the water it looks clean and clear. However when you stir it the mud from the bottom is brought to the surface making the water cloudy and muddy. If you remove the mud floating on the surface the stream will appear to be clear although some mud will have sunk back down to the bottom. Repeating this process enough times the muddy stream will eventually be reborn as a clear one.

By the same process Reiki stirs and removes toxins from our system. After receiving Reiki treatment, initially a person's condition may appear to become worse but this should not be seen as a problem. It is merely a part of the natural cleansing process.

The Finest Paper ...

Hayashi Sensei also used another metaphor. The effects of Reiki are like slowly peeling off sheets of the finest paper, so it is important to continue until recovery is complete. For acute problems the immediate effects of Reiki are easy to see. However, chronic illness, although it takes more time, can be cured too. Once you become able to feel *Byosen* (troubled areas) you will agree that the effects of Reiki are like slowly and gently peeling off sheets of the finest paper until the healthy being is revealed.

Byosen—Feeling the Troubled Areas

In the afternoon of this first seminar they switched to practical training on how to give a Reiki treatment. They used a type of rattan bed called "Reiki tables" which were 40 cm high, just the right height for those giving a Reiki treatment whilst sitting on the floor.

There were several tables but when necessary futons (Japanese style bedding mats) were used to accommodate extra people. The practical training session was a very enthusiastic one. The participants were able to receive a treatment themselves and had the chance to practice their freshly learned Reiki on people in poor health.

Hayashi Sensei also gave them practical instructions as to how to recognize *Byosen*. Chiyoko was able to feel *it* quite easily. She was very excited at the prospect of understanding what *it* was really like because she had heard the word so frequently. She still remembers clearly how intently the other participants tried to recognize *it*.

The instructions were as follows: While practicing Reiki on a patient your hands may feel unusual sensations in certain body areas. This is called *Byosen* ("byo" means ill, stiffness or tumor, "sen" means gland).

Byosen has its peaks and troughs and is divided into five levels:

1. *Warmth*	heat slightly higher than body temperature.
2. *Strong heat*	more intense heat.
3. *Tingling*	a tingling sensation in the hands or fingers which becomes increasingly strong until it peaks out and slowly becomes weaker. During one treatment of 30-50 min it will peak about 3 times. It is as if you are repeatedly climbing a mountain. It becomes easier each time. The patient should start to feel better at this point.
4. *Pulse-like sensation*	*Hibiki* or a pulse-like feeling in your hands indicates that you can actually feel the Reiki stimulating blood vessels, causing them to expand and contract. At this time the blood circulation is activated and the blood begins to flow more smoothly.
5. *Pain*	tells the practitioner that the *Byosen* is serious. The more painful your hands the more serious the prob-

lem is. Pain can move from your palm to the back of your hand, to your wrist and gradually to around the elbow area. Sometimes it stops there and other times it may move up to your shoulder. After the pain eases the tingling sensation decreases also.

When experiencing this pain some people may become worried about receiving negative energy from the patient but this is not possible so do not worry unnecessarily. Taking your hands off the patient can easily relieve this pain although it occasionally continues for a short time.

Hayashi Sensei encouraged everybody to practice in order to make their hands more sensitive to *Byosen*. He taught it at the seminars through actual practice. To feel *Byosen* is a key element for a Reiki practitioner. With practice it becomes easy to feel *Byosen* while giving a Reiki treatment.

The second day of the seminar consisted of *Reiju, Reiki Mawashi* (Reiki circulation), practical lessons on how to make the hands more sensitive plus an actual Reiki treatment session. This was followed by lectures using an anatomical chart to give understanding of the functions of each organ and application of Reiki depending on a person's symptoms.

The 5 days passed really quickly and Chiyoko's dream had been realized. She then attended seminars every month including the special ones when Hayashi Sensei came each Spring and Autumn. She practiced at home almost everyday.

The Reiki Practice after Her First Seminar

Both Usui Sensei and Hayashi Sensei placed more importance on practice than on theory. Chiyoko appreciated this because it was much easier for her to understand. What she learned at the seminar was quite familiar to her already because it was exactly what she had always heard from her uncle, aunt and sister when they gave Reiki treatments to their patients. After the seminar she re-read her notes often and reviewed with her family what she had learned. She clearly remembers the entire contents of the seminars which makes this material wholly available for people who attend the seminars we hold today.

Chiyoko started her actual treatments at home for those in need around her. Her sister, Katsue, already had a good reputation for her Reiki and many people came to her for treatments. Some even came to pick her up by car to take her to a patient's home.

Their mother was happy to see her daughters being kind and helping others, so she truly appreciated Mr. Sugano bringing Reiki into the family. She did every thing she could to make it easy for her daughters to give Reiki treatments, serving their patients tea and creating a relaxed atmosphere in the house. In those days Reiki was performed purely as a social service and not as a business.

The Remarkable Results of Reiki

Here is one amazing story from Chiyoko.

In her neighborhood there was a 3-year-old boy who had burned his hand while he was alone at home. Playing by the fire he had accidentally burnt himself and the resulting injury was really serious covering his entire hand. It was only a few days later that he was brought to Chiyoko. The burn had started to fester and his hand had turned bright yellow. Chiyoko still remembers the terrible smell. The boy's mother told them that he had not been able sleep at night because of the pain. It was so serious that when she first looked at it Chiyoko was not sure if she could help him.

Together with her sister and aunt she gave the boy a Reiki treatment and to their surprise he fell asleep within 20 or 30 minutes. This encouraged Chiyoko to keep going. They gave him Reiki every day and by the third day the weeping on his hand had eased. After 5 days the burns had visibly improved. Several days later the surface of the burnt skin peeled off like a snake shedding its skin. Underneath fresh skin and fingernails were beginning to regenerate. His fingers started to function normally and it took only a short time to see a great recovery. The boy's parents were delighted and both Chiyoko and the others who had been able to help him with Reiki were truly impressed.

There was a second case in her neighborhood in which a boy with less serious burns had received conventional medical treatment from a doctor. His fingers became stuck to the palm of his hand and he ended up having an operation to amputate the ends of his fingers. Such experiences made Chiyoko more certain about the great benefits of Reiki treatment and she enjoyed practicing it more and more. She remembers those days clearly, and always describes them vividly.

Reiki during the Second World War

By 1938 there were already around 450 Reiki practitioners in Daishoji and Osaka. Among them some, including Chiyoko's uncle, aunt and sister, held *Shihankaku* and *Shihan* degrees. It had been 10 years since her uncle Mr. Sugano had first learned Reiki in Osaka. Chiyoko was granted *Shihankaku* degree in the Spring of 1939 and *Shihan* degree that Autumn. She achieved these degrees much more quickly than usual because of her deep association with Reiki and close connection to Hayashi Sensei through Mr. Sugano.

Her uncle had chosen Shonosuke Yamaguchi as her future husband and decided to send him to the Manchurian branch of his company as a CEO. Mr. Sugano was quite certain that there would be a war and knew that Reiki would be needed in Manchuria (then a colony of Japan).

Chiyoko was married in 1942 and stayed in Manchuria until the war ended. Throughout good times and bad Reiki helped her and enabled her to help others which was greatly appreciated by everyone involved. She is still very grateful to Hayashi Sensei and to her uncle Mr. Sugano for opening the way for her to help so many people.

The Facts Surrounding Hayashi Sensei's Death

How Hayashi Sensei died is thought to be a mystery but the facts are known.

A relative of Chiyoko Yamaguchi heard the story directly from Chie Hayashi, Hayashi Sensei's wife.

The war was becoming increasingly fierce and as an ex-serviceman Hayashi Sensei was expecting imminent call up for military service. Having become a dedicated practitioner of Reiki under the instruction of Usui Sensei it was impossible for him to participate in the war as a military officer, even as a medical officer. He knew that he would not be permitted to provide Reiki treatments on the battlefield and that he would have to practice conventional medicine with which he did not agree.

Because of his travel to Hawaii Hayashi Sensei was also suspected of being a spy. He was faced with the impossible choice between going to war or being imprisoned and executed. He decided to die with dignity and ended his life himself in the presence of his wife and some of his students.

After Hayashi Sensei's Death

Upon his death Mrs. Chie Hayashi succeeded her husband in conducting the Hayashi Reiki Kenkyu-kai (seminars) and traveled Japan in her husband's place. She visited the Daishoji branch several times each year for *Reiju-Kai* (attunement sessions).

In 1941 some members of the Daishoji branch held a Buddhist memorial ceremony for Hayashi Sensei and since then such ceremonies have been held on several occasions. Even at times when Mrs. Hayashi did not come to Daishoji *Reiju-kai* continued under the initiative of some *Shihan*s until 1950 when she began to visit more frequently.

Almost all the people who attended those seminars with Chie Hayashi Sensei have passed away so it has been difficult to ascertain the exact details. Only snippets of those times survive. One person remembers that at the memorial service for Hayashi Sensei in 1952 a lady called Mrs. Takata came from Hawaii to pay her respects. Chie Hayashi Sensei asked her to come to Japan permanently and to take over Hayashi Reiki Kenkyu-kai but she declined. It had been too long since she had learned Reiki from Hayashi Sensei and she had already started to alter and popularize it in Hawaii. It is not certain how seriously Mrs. Hayashi tried to convince Mrs. Takata to accept her proposal but she often lamented the difficulties in finding suitable successors.

Today there are quite a few Reiki practitioners in Japan but they are not actively promoting this original style of Reiki.

We have now established *Jikiden Reiki* Seminars in order to preserve the original ideas and lineage of Usui Sensei and Hayashi Sensei. We hope *Jikiden Reiki* will empower people all over the world enabling them to reawaken their natural healing abilities and ultimately create a healthier society.

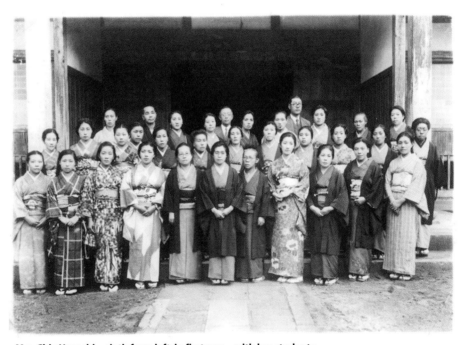

Mrs. Chie Hayashi—sixth from left, in first row—with her students

Chapter 3

An Interesting Reiki Article from 1928

The following is an article published on March 4th 1928 in "SUNDAY MAINICHI", a widely circulated magazine in Japan. It was written by Mr. Shou Matsui (1870-1933) in response to readers' questions and gives some idea of how people thought about medicine at the time.

Mr. Matsui was born in Miyazaki (Southern Japan) and worked for the Chuo and Hochi Newspapers (in 1885 & 1886 respectively) before entering the theatrical world. Known as a playwright and a teacher of acting he had made a major contribution to traditional Japanese Kabuki theatre and was acquainted with a large number of Kabuki actors. After studying Reiki Ryoho under Chujiro Hayashi Sensei he conveyed his enthusiasm for Reiki to many of the actors who as a result themselves went on to learn Reiki.

The article reads (printed originally in Japanese):

I would love to answer your questions readers:

This treatment, which can cure all kinds of diseases is known as "Reiki

Ryoho" and is practiced by an exclusive group of people. It's founder or creator, Dr. Mikao Usui passed away a few years ago. His students now practice in their own clinics and continue to initiate others into Reiki Ryoho. Unfortunately, despite the remarkable effectiveness of this style of treatment, Dr. Usui was not fond of advertising Reiki and consequently his students hesitate to publicize it either. As a result Reiki is not yet well known.

Nevertheless, I would like to be the one to publicize it in order to help the larger population. I feel particularly obliged to answer the questions asked by "DAIMAI TONICHI", a widely circulated newspaper. I wish to prevent journalists and readers from thinking that Reiki Ryoho is a sham because it seems as though the people involved are claiming they can't tell you anything as they don't like promulgating their methods!

It is reasonable to assume that people might choose not to make any medical claims in order to avoid being held responsible in case of failure. However, I'm going to take the risk and the responsibility in order to publicize the truth about Reiki. For Reiki's

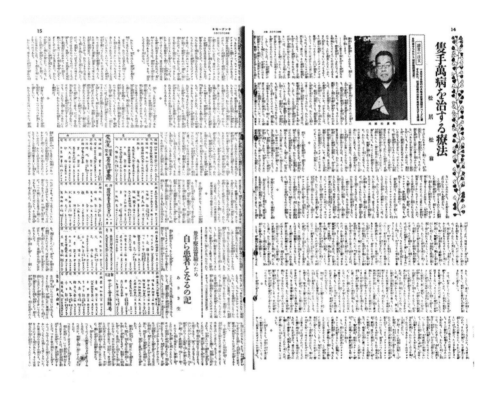

隻手萬病を治する療法

松居松翁

sake and the sake of people suffering from ill health I just cannot hold my tongue, so I am acting alone when I write this. And as it has nothing to do with other Reiki practitioners I will take sole responsibility for my words. I myself am so excited about this treatment that I haven't been able to concentrate on my usual work of writing scripts for plays since I first learned it.

When I can propagate it effectively and my goal of an ideal world is realized, Japanese people will be a great deal happier. Moreover people all over the world will be in excellent health. I just want to introduce this amazing thing to everyone!

From this article you can see that Mr. Matsui was extremely frustrated with Usui Sensei and Hayashi Sensei's attitudes towards the promotion of Reiki. Despite its effectiveness Usui Sensei clearly did not want to propagate Reiki, believing instead that it should be circulated by word of mouth to those who would fully understand it and use it effectively. Genuine things need not be broadcast loudly to survive and so Reiki has been popularized in this manner until recently.

The following section of the article concerns Hayashi Sensei himself:

It has been more than 10 years since Reiki Ryoho was founded however there have only been a few clinics established to provide Reiki treatments. Chujiro Hayashi, a diligent warm-hearted naval captain who looks as if he was born to be a Reiki practitioner initiated me into Reiki. Hayashi Sensei gives Reiki treatments to patients in the mornings and holds seminars 5 days a month to initiate new people into Reiki.

The problem is that there are a number of other styles of treatment (which appear to be bogus) with the Chinese character "Rei" in their name and people often wrongly associate Reiki with such sects. Despite this, Hayashi Sensei is not willing to speak out to differentiate Reiki from these factions so I guess it's natural that his great style of Reiki treatment is not practiced as widely as is needed.

I would like to clarify that Reiki is the most unique and successful treatment for all ailments, at least for all those I have ever come across. You may wonder if Reiki can help those with psychological problems. It can. It produces amazing results on every conceivable problem both internally and externally, On intestinal disorders, external injuries, burns, rheumatism and nervous breakdowns to name but a few! In short, it really works whatever the problem!

Mr. Matsui practiced Reiki on more than 100 people in a short period of time. He became increasingly convinced of its effectiveness each time he saw the incredible results. He goes on to talk about a few of his experiences:

Let me give you examples rather than theory:

A recent example is that of a 4-year-old girl brought to me by her father who had heard about me by word of mouth. The little girl had lost the sight in one eye and her remaining eye was becoming infected. They had visited a great number of doctors for help but had been told that nothing could be done for her. In desperation, they finally came to me. I suspected that there would be problems in other areas of her body and so I examined her fully and discovered that the disease was causing difficulties all over her body—her stomach, intestines, nose and kidneys. However the visible symptoms had manifested in her eyes.

I gave her Reiki treatment and after 5 or 6 sessions her eyesight started to return and her other symptoms also gradually improved. Her devoted father kept saying that he would not have minded giving his own eyes to help his daughter. As a result he chose to learn Reiki in order to continue to heal her.

The following case occurred last December. "Mr. O", a well-known artist, was on the verge of death. His doctor had told his family that he had approximately 3 hours to live. When the family contacted me it was midnight and 2 hours had already passed. My wife and I drove quickly to his home in a suburb of Tokyo. It took an hour and a half to get there and when we arrived, his family were waiting anxiously at the front gate. They told us that he had had a heart attack as the result of vascular disease.

We immediately laid our hands on his heart and gave him Reiki continuously for 6 hours straight without even stopping for a sip of tea. After this time his doctor told us that his heartbeat, which had been dangerously fast, had returned to a safe rhythm. The following day his temperature returned to normal and his pulse held at about 80. I would like to proclaim that it is not so hard to lower a person's heartbeat from 120 to 80 within a few hours with Reiki.

Last but not least Mr. Kichisaburo who had 4 great doctors tell him that he was going to die. At the very last moment as his family were saying goodbye to him I was there to try to bring him back. He survived!

There are countless miraculous stories like these. However nothing is actually miraculous, quite simply these people received a practical treatment, which activates the body's natural healing process.

Lastly Mr. Matsui explains a little about how easy it is to become a Reiki practitioner:

A mutual friend introduced me to Mr. Hayashi and I decided to learn Reiki from him. I paid a fortune to be attuned. There are different levels of study, Shoden and Okuden are two of them. I have learned Shoden level but am still a beginner so as yet I haven't been ready to move to the Okuden level. I don't know all the details yet but I have noticed that there seems to be a hierarchy among the students. I find it quite interesting that these well-intentioned people, who are too modest to brag about the wonderful things they can do, have created such a hierarchy and charge so much money for giving initiations. However I do believe that they should be allowed to maintain their own interests. But I feel so frustrated that I am not free to talk about the details of the initiation and treatment. In my opinion it is a great loss for everyone.

I am at least able to tell you that if you learn Reiki for an hour and a half each day for 5 days you will be able to give treatments to people. Some people can give them from the very first day. It really is easy to learn. All humans possess a subconscious which is activated as a sixth sense by Reiki during these 5 days. From that time simply by laying your hands on problematic areas of the body the treatment starts. I don't think there is a treatment method more simple than this. I so want to make this available to everyone not only to the wealthy. Unfortunately I am not permitted to do that because Medical Law forbids unconventional treatment. I will however endeavor to let as many people as possible know about this fantastic treatment.

At that time Western medicine was already the mainstream. With the exception of certain traditional Oriental medicines other medical treatments were in violation of Medical Law. There were alternative treatment styles other than Reiki but most practitioners gave up when challenged by the accepted Oriental medical practitioners who informed on them.

Reiki was particularly threatening because it is so easy and effective. Hence it was spread only by word of mouth among those who could be trusted not to talk about it in the wrong places. These people were so convinced by its effectiveness that they were willing to pay a great deal of money to learn it. Mr. Matsui was taking a big risk introducing the results of such treatments into the public domain.

Some of the groups outlawed at that time evolved as religious groups that still exist today. Their styles transformed from treatments into the practice of religious prayer rituals. Obviously Reiki has also survived in its original form. However, in today's Japan ideas about alternative medicine remain largely unchanged.

Mr. Matsui who practiced Reiki without payment wrote this article around the same time as Chiyoko's uncle Wasaburo Sugano Sensei was learning Reiki. Both Mr. Matsui's article and Sugano Sensei's story illustrate how Reiki began to become known as a highly effective treatment for all kinds of problems.

The *Jikiden Reiki* group continues to give effective treatments and is endeavoring to actively promote Reiki. In doing so we are seeking to contribute to realizing Mr. Matsui's dream of a world in which everyone can benefit from good health.

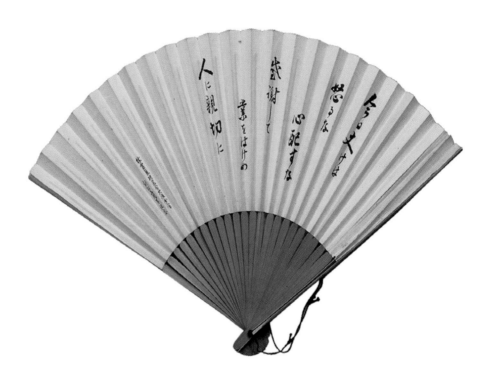

Japanese fan stamped with the Reiki Life Principles, handwritten by Dr. Hayashi—for the fifth anniversary of *Hayashi Reiki Kenkyu-Kai* (The Hayashi Reiki Practice Group)

Practical Part

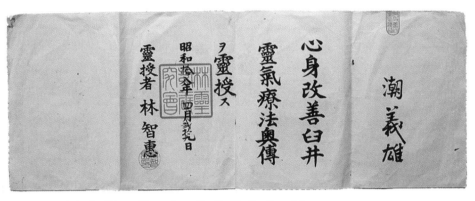

Another original Reiki certificate signed by Dr. Chujiro Hayashi

Chapter 4

Byosen and Ketsueki Kokan (Blood Circulation Technique)

Byosen

The Japanese and Western Reiki schools differ in one central way. In Western Reiki we are taught that Reiki is "intelligent" and that it will find its way to the areas in the body that need it the most. Of course this seems true but it is only half the truth. The other half is that the body wants Reiki and will let the practitioner know where and how it wants to be touched. This happens through what Japanese Reiki practitioners call "*Byosen*".

This concept is new to many of us and because it takes such a vital role in Japanese Reiki, I would like to elaborate on it further.

In Dr. Usui's original group, the Usui Reiki Ryoho Gakkai, the ability to perceive the *Byosen* was a prerequisite to the student advancing to the Second Reiki Degree. In Dr. Hayashi's system it is held that this ability is absolutely necessary in order to be able to help the client's body heal itself.

As Tadao has already mentioned in Chapter 2 the *Byosen* is perceived either as warmth, strong heat, tingling, a pulsating feeling in the hands or as pain. I would describe the *Byosen* as "tension".

This tension develops around disease in the body and is easily felt by the practitioner. You may feel either one or a variety of the aforementioned sensations, a tingle in your hands, excess heat or cold, a magnetic pull or push, or "pins and needles" piercing your hands. This feeling is not "bad", it is simply the way the client's body tells the practitioner where his hands are most needed. Be grateful for the hint!

When touching a problem area you may feel pain in your hands. If the disease is serious the pain may travel up to your elbows or even up to your shoulders. If it is bearable keep your hands on the afflicted area until it traces back down and leaves your hands. This does not mean that you are taking the client's pain into your own body. It is simply a natural process that needs to go through its stages. If the pain is too intense take your hands off the body and shake them out several times before replacing them to recommence the treatment.

It is possible that the art of sensing the *Byosen* was deleted from of the Western Reiki practice by Mrs. Takata and her students because it implies a certain kind of diagnosis.

In most countries it is not permitted to make a medical diagnosis unless one is a licensed health-care practitioner. If you are a Reiki practitioner who is not licensed you may get into serious trouble with the law if you share what you feel with your clients. So if a diagnosis should come to you keep it to yourself or share it with your client in a discreet manner. Make sure that you are well informed about the medical laws where you are practicing. The answer to this challenge may lie in obtaining a Homeopathic Doctor's license, a Massage Practitioner or Chiropractor license.

The best way to deal with this issue if you are not licensed is to have your patients sign an agreement before you begin with the treatment. They must sign that they are taking your treatment of their own accord, that they take sole responsibility for the results and that they are aware of the fact that this is not a medical treatment. Check the legal requirements for this protection with a local lawyer.

If you feel that your client is seriously ill you must suggest to him to go and see a physician. Be careful with the way you package this information. If you tell a client that he has probably a serious heart problem you may make the condition worse. Can you imagine the effect of a physician telling his patient that his heart is beyond repair? A diagnosis of this sort is like a death sentence! We need to consider the power of the words we use very carefully. We need to think about the effect of our statements and in some cases this means that silence is golden.

When treating life threatening illnesses the *Byosen* may make itself felt during the whole treatment and beyond. Best would be to keep your hands on the body part that displays the *Byosen* but this may not be possible.

Treat the person daily for at least an hour, more if possible and get extra help from other Reiki practitioners if you can. With life threatening illnesses several hours of Reiki per day may make the difference. Your hands may not move at all for the whole duration of the treatment. If that happens stay where you feel the *Byosen* and come back to the same area next time you see your client.

On the one hand you are responsible for sharing what you feel because your client may depend upon it. On the other hand you have to learn to package your understanding in a way that is neither a diagnosis nor a prophecy. You could tell your client that it would be good for him to have his internal organs checked out medically. You can tell him that it is a good thing to do every once in a while. You may even tell him that you yourself have done it recently …

Western medical science has not been able to solve one very common riddle. They call it "spontaneous remission". Almost ten percent of all cancer patients encounter this remission. This suggests that science does not know why either sickness or healing occur.

There is no such thing as an incurable disease. The miracle of life is cradled in the hands of the divine.

The Attire of the Practitioner

It is important to avoid resembling a physician. No need for a white doctor's jacket nor medical charts on the walls of your session room, and it's important not to give your clients any medical advice.

It is also important not to suggest taking or reducing any medication. If your client is in psychiatric treatment ask him first to discuss the proposed Reiki treatment with his psychiatrist. A good way of working is to collaborate closely with a physician.

Feeling the Byosen—Exercises

To get a clear feeling for the *Byosen* practice the following exercise with a partner.

Byosen Partner Exercises

Place one hand on your own knee or thigh (if they are healthy, otherwise choose another non-tense part of the body) and the other one on the shoulder of your partner in front of you.

Feel the difference of perception in each of your hands. The hand resting on your knee will feel "normal". It may feel warm and relaxed, radiating energy in a calm and even manner, the same way you perceive a "normal" pulse. The other hand will feel the tension in your partner's shoulders and upper back. Since most of us lead rather sedentary lives and have acquired poor posture we have tense shoulders. Through this exercise you will be able to recognize the difference between a relaxed and harmonious part of the body and a tense one.

Keep your hand on your partner's shoulders for a few minutes and give him Reiki. The sensation of the Byosen will become less intense as you go along.

If the tension is not very pronounced in the first place it may even vanish all together and your partner will be enveloped in warmth and relaxation.

Now switch your hands.

The sensitivity of your right and left hands is likely to be slightly different. It is not a question of being right or left-handed. For some right handers the left hand is more sensitive than the right and vice versa. Experiment and find out for yourself: is it the Byosen that you feel or is it the energy in your own hand?

For example, if you have one hand under the back of a large client, the pulse that you feel may be the circulation problem in your own hand caused by your client's body weight! So experiment with switching hands. Which hand is more sensitive? If there is a noticeable difference you may wish to bring more sensitivity to the less sensitive hand. If for a while you use this hand predominantly when treating your clients it will become equally sensitive.

The Attitude of a Practitioner towards His Client's Suffering

It is natural to feel empathy with your clients. You may feel their physical, emotional or mental pain, or a mixture of these. Tears may come to your eyes and your heart may ache. This is absolutely natural.

Just remember one thing: don't make your client's pain your own. It is important to learn the art of letting go.

Practice this experiment with these rituals.

1. After your client has gone say to yourself: "I am letting go of your pain and suffering. It is not mine." Or, "I trust that healing has been set in motion."

2. Practice a self-cleansing ritual before and after each treatment. Wash your hands with cold water up to the elbows, gargle and go to the toilet if possible. Drink a glass of mineral water. If you know them use one of Dr. Usui's "kenyoku" techniques described in "The Spirit of Reiki"*.

---

* Lübeck/Petter/Rand: *The Spirit of Reiki*, Lotus Press, Twin Lakes, WI, 2001, page 153f.

3. Go on a "mental fast". Stop thinking or worrying about your client and his suffering, however severe it may be, the moment he leaves your premises. Every time the thought of him comes up remind yourself to let it go, with love.

Observing Silently and Accurately

Because we have the capacity to empathize with one another a diagnosis is a natural occurrence. During a Reiki treatment your heart is wide open and you feel or sense what is going on with your client. This knowledge may show itself in five different ways, depending on your type and skill. Some of us are predominantly body, mind, or spirit centered and the area of your predominance is the one that you are likely to encounter more strongly.

1. The Physical Level

When you touch the body of your client it may tell you what physically ails it. You may be able to "look" into her body. You may see or feel blocked up arteries, a cyst in the womb, or the toxicity of your client's blood.

Don't be surprised if you see the body from the inside, even though your knowledge of physiology may be limited. Get a good book on human anatomy and study it carefully. Many years ago I met a healer in Austria who could "test" the blood of his clients with the accuracy of a laboratory. This may sound far-fetched to you but... everything is possible. You do not need to be a psychic or an incredibly advanced spiritual being to develop such skills. All of us are borne with divine gifts. Learn to accept them and put them into practice.

2. The Energetic Level

You may make an energetic diagnosis of your client and find that there is an etheric deficiency in one of the organs. You may feel his meridians and his chakras. Get some literature on the meridian and chakra systems and compare the knowledge you find there with your own insights. Be ready to experiment and trust yourself.

You may feel that the energy is not moving well through one of the meridians, the chakras or the etheric body. You may feel you know what your client needs to do in order to harmonize his energy body with exercises, diet or mental work. Trust this.

It is also possible that a client may experience spontaneous memories of past lives during a Reiki treatment. Physics tell us that no energy is ever lost. This also holds true for the energy of thought and emotion. Memories are thoughts and they may reappear during a Reiki treatment when the client is in an altered state of mind.

The way I see reincarnation it is transpersonal. Imagine a wave in the ocean. It is lifted up above the surface of the waters temporarily before it dissolves into whole again. A moment later another wave grows above the waters. Who is to say that the first and the second wave are different waves? They are made of the same water.…. In this light reincarnation and the memories of past lives are not such far out ideas.

3. The Psychological Level

You may perceive your client's psychological difficulties. You may "see" or feel his mother or his father before your eyes. Perhaps when you touched his physical form in the past you suddenly saw your client at the age of three or four. If it happens again ask him if he went through a traumatic experience at that time in his life and if he wants to share what torments his heart with you. A whole tidal wave of emotional healing may now roll in.

The most important attitude for a practitioner in such cases is to remain the unidentified witness, not judging what you hear, not organizing what your client shares with you into moral boxes of good and bad. Become all ears! Milton Erickson, the founder of modern Hypnotherapy suggested that a counselor should imagine himself floating up above the client and himself to a "meta position" from where he can see the whole picture and help the client find a solution best for all people involved.

If you are not prepared to carry out psychological work refer your client to a psychologist or to a professional counselor.

4. The Emotional Level

You may cry with your client. Enjoy it! This does not mean that you are taking his suffering as your own. Feel it and get it over with. This happens to me very often and I appreciate the depth the tears bring with them … for a while.

You may feel certain emotions that have lodged themselves into the client's muscle tissue. Whenever these body areas are stimulated by touch the emotions can break loose. Afterwards your client may need continuing emotional support.

Generally speaking it is helpful to encourage a client to express his emotions during a Reiki treatment. Don't worry. Help him to allow whatever is locked in the body to come out. Hidden traumas may well heal in the light of expression. But expression is double edged. It can strengthen a client or weaken him.

You will be able to distinguish between a strengthening and a weakening emotion when you touch the client's body. Emotional pain has a beautiful depth and can be used as an agent for healing. If you feel that the client is getting lost in self-pity or guilty feelings, which are emotional dreams, ask him to open his eyes and to look into yours. With this intervention you bring him back to this moment, where time stands still.

5. The Spiritual Level

A spiritual diagnosis is the most difficult to make and I personally have no experience in this. The spiritual goes far beyond what can be grasped with the mind and extreme caution needs be exercised when tempted to assess what cannot be assessed. If your client experiences a spiritual phenomenon or a spiritual crisis during a treatment find someone who can support him afterwards. You may know a spiritual master or teacher who can be contacted in your area.

Perception Training

Perception training is everything. An ancient Tantric Hindu meditation says that wherever attention alights the energy increases. You can prove this statement for yourself with a simple experiment. Close your eyes for a moment and take a couple of deep breaths. Let go of the tensions of the past and relax into the present moment. Feel your body, your breath and become intensely aware of where you are right now.

Now pay attention to the tip of the little finger on your left hand and forget everything else. Feel it for a few moments and then begin to increase the energy in it. Imagine the Reiki energy moving in the direction of your pinky and then filling it. Now feel how it radiates from your little finger. It may suddenly feel huge or you may see it filled with light and energy. When you feel it pulsating with Reiki energy place it on a part of your own body that needs love and attention. You will be surprised how powerful this little finger has become. You can work only with what you are aware of.

The First Steps to Learn Byosen

To train the sensitivity of your hands practice this exercise:

Feel the Energy

Rub your hands gently together for one minute and pay attention to the heat and energy that the rubbing sets free. Now move your hands apart very slowly and gently until they are one inch from each other. Do you feel the energy between your hands? Do you feel the heat, or a tingling, or a magnetic pull? Stay with this for a moment and then move your hands farther from each other. Stop again for a minute or two when they are two inches apart, then continue drawing them farther apart. Every time you feel the distance has grown too much stop and feel. When you reach a point where you can't feel the energy between your hands any more stop and move them closer together again. Stop for a moment and feel. Now move them closer together once more, in slow motion. Stop again and feel and then move them yet closer together until the palms touch each other. Remain with the palms touching in the *Gassho* position for a few minutes. Feel how you have both energized and sensitized your hands.

Do this exercise regularly …

When you feel familiar with the Reiki energy in your hands practice this with another Reiki practitioner.

Feel the Energy while Sitting Together

Sit opposite one another and place the palms of your hands against those of your partner. After a minute or so move your hands one inch apart. Continue as in the exercise above moving farther and farther away from your partner's hands, stopping every once in a while. Finish off by coming closer and closer to your partner again until the palms of your hands are touching. Remain with your palms touching each other for a couple of minutes.

Feel the Energy while Standing Together

The next time you work with your partner start out by standing opposite one another with your palms touching. Now move slowly away from each other creating a distance of about three feet. Extend both hands with the palms facing your partner and feel his energy. Feel the space that divides the two of you and feel where your energy body touches his. As you practice move farther and farther away from your partner. Every time you feel a change in your perception stop and feel. If you come to a point where you can't feel your partner any more stop and come a little closer together until the connection is re-established. From this point on move slowly towards your partner until the palms of your hands touch

Feel the Energy Together at a Greater Distance

The next time you practice, experiment to see if you can move still farther apart and yet feel your partner. Practice until you are standing on one side of the room and your partner on the other. To end this exercise come slowly closer together until your palms touch one another.

Now that you know how to feel the energy of people, experiment with animals and plants. After you have practiced this for a while move on to inanimate objects. Take an apple in your hands and feel its energy. Feel its vitality. Feel the tree it has grown on and the place in which it grew. Feel the sun and the moon that have shone upon it, the rain and the nutrients that have nourished it. Now feel whether this apple is good for you. Practice this with all the foods you eat. Are fruits and vegetables good for you? What about seafood and meat, milk products and grains? What about drinks and sweets?

Advanced Techniques

Several years ago I noticed that I could sense my clients' bodies from the "inside". This brought the understanding of the Byosen one step further. The first time it happened I was holding the client's feet lightly, touching the inside of both feet just below the ankle with the index, middle and ring fingers of both hands. I suddenly perceived my client's whole body at once, the same way you feel the whole form of an apple if you wrap your hands around it. I felt not only the outside of his body but the inside as well. I could feel his feet, his legs, his inner organs, his back, his head, his hair... I could feel where the energy was moving freely and where it was obstructed. The problem areas felt like dark spots in a light-body, like dark holes in the Milky Way.

My client confirmed what I had felt and I began paying attention to the people I work with in this new way.

This journey has become of great value for me personally because it has helped me to acquire the right orientation on this path. I realized that I could only work in this way if I was in a certain meditative state of mind. This state does not require sitting quietly for hours prior to the treatment or becoming a great yogi. The first ingredient is single-pointedness. When you touch your client be totally there for him and don't allow your mind to wander off somewhere else. Be one hundred percent present. Be one hundred percent touch! Give the client everything you have, allowing a space of unconditional love. He is perfect the way he is, even if he is very ill. This moment is all that counts, only in this moment is life happening...

It has been my experience that internal scanning can happen while touching any part of the client's body. However there are four areas of the body that make it especially easy for someone who has not done it before.

1. Scanning below the ankles
Place the fingers of both hands below your client's ankles in the indentation between the ankle and the heel. Curl your fingers lightly so your fingertips rest on the client's feet. The fingertips are extremely sensitive because they are homes to many nerves and the end points of the major meridians. Practicing in this fashion is a good way to make them more sensitive. Many of us have learned to apply Reiki with the palms of the hands only and this will add a great deal of pleasure to your work. Apply a little bit of pressure, as much as it takes to depress the skin slightly, and keep your hands on this place without moving.

2. Scanning in the Medulla Oblongata
Ask your client to lie on his back. When he has found a comfortable position slide your hands under his head and place your fingers under his medulla oblongata (where the spine enters the skull). Curl your fingers lightly and allow them to rest there without moving.

3. Scanning on the Temples
Place both of your hands on the client's temples in a way that your curled fingertips rest behind the client's eyes.

4. Scanning the Touching of the Hands
Place your fingertips in the center of your client's palms. Curl them a little and let them rest there without moving. As an alternative take one or both of your client's hands into yours and hold.

Preliminary Scanning Exercises

Before you set out to scan the body of a client from the inside practice with your own body.

Feel the Totality

Lie down and close your eyes for ten minutes having made sure that you will not be disturbed during this time. Feel your own body from the inside. For now don't pay attention to separate parts of the body. Feel the whole "bag of skin" as one. You may either get an inner "image" of your body or you may feel it in its entirety.

Go into the Detail

Lie down and close your eyes for ten minutes having made sure that you will not be disturbed. In this exercise you will go through your own body sending your consciousness into every part, one at a time. Start with your dominant hand. Feel every finger, beginning with the thumb and then moving from the index finger to the middle finger, the ring finger and on to the pinky. Now feel the palm of your hand, the back of your hand and your wrist, then the whole hand as one unit. Repeat this with your non-dominant hand.

Move back to your dominant arm and feel it from the wrist to the forearm, then from the elbow to the shoulder. Do the same with the non-dominant arm.

Now move to your right leg, then the left leg and so on until you have covered your whole body.

Give yourself ten minutes before you jump into the "real world" again.

Internal Scanning

I have found two ways of approaching the art of inner scanning. The one that came to me first was to perceive the whole body at once, in its entirety. When you look at an object, unless it is extremely complex, your mind is able to perceive and understand it completely. You know an apple or a desk wholly when you look at it. The same skill can be learned when looking at a client. The human mind is used to compartmentalizing the complex objects that it sees in order not to feel overwhelmed. We pick apart what we see into small and understandable pieces. You may look at your client's head and mentally sever it from the rest of the body. This may be a useful tool when in conversation but when treating a person it is more helpful to see him in his totality. Body, mind and soul are one unit and they need to be treated as such.

Internal Scanning—Perceiving the Body as a Whole

When you first meet your client shake hands paying close attention to whatever you feel. Is his hand-shake strong, weak, confident, insecure, warm or cold? Immediately you will acquire non-verbal information about your client that you could not gather from conversation. Look into his eyes and pay attention to his skin tone, his breathing and his movements. Are they soft and gentle or hard and abrupt. How does he walk and how does he sit down? Is he focussed or absent minded? Is he in emotional turmoil or calm and collected? Ask him your standard questions about his life and lifestyle and why he has come to see you.

When he is lying down look at the way his body is lying there. Are his shoulders the same height? Does one come up higher than the other? How is the position of his head and neck? Do both legs appear to have the same length and do they rest in the same position? All this will give you information about the general state of his body and his mind.

Record whatever you see and feel in your mind and then begin with the scanning. First place both hands in the manner described above on any one of the five body areas suggested.

Perceive your client's body as one unit that cannot be divided into different parts. Feel it in its entirety.

Inner Scanning—Analyzing All the Parts

Now to the second technique. To practice this successfully it will help to have some knowledge of anatomy. If you are insecure about your knowledge obtain a good book on human anatomy and study it before using this technique.

Begin by placing both hands in the manner described above on any one of the four parts of the body suggested. Now let your consciousness enter the head of the client and feel it from the inside.

Feel the brain in its complexity. Feel its thoughts and its emptiness. Feel both its halves and their functions, the rational and the intuitive, the linear and the abstract. Feel the anatomy of the brain. What does it look like? Do you see or sense any blocks? Do you sense destructive thought patterns? If yes record them in your memory or write them down and share them with your client later should this seem appropriate.

Now move on to feel the eyes, the ears, the nasal cavity, the sinuses and so on. Feel every part of the body without allowing your mind to wander elsewhere. After you have scanned the client's head from the inside move down and scan the throat. Continue with the chest and back, the vital organs, the abdomen and lower back and finally the legs and feet.

The Breath of Heaven and Earth

When you have practiced the two techniques above and feel comfortable with them add further spice to your treatment. Your clients will love your hands!

The Breath

Sit comfortably with both of your feet on the ground. Take a few breaths and leave past and future behind. Be Here and Now. Breathe in through your nose, through the crown chakra and the soles of your feet all at the same time. Pull the breath all the way down into your Tanden (Chinese, Dantien, two or three fingers below the navel).

While breathing in imagine that you are bringing in the energy of Heaven through your crown chakra and the energy of the Earth through your soles. Hold the breath in your Dantien for a few seconds and then breathe out through your mouth. As you breathe out imagine that the energy of the Heavens and the energy of the Earth are flowing into your client's body, nourishing him with the universal life force, Reiki!

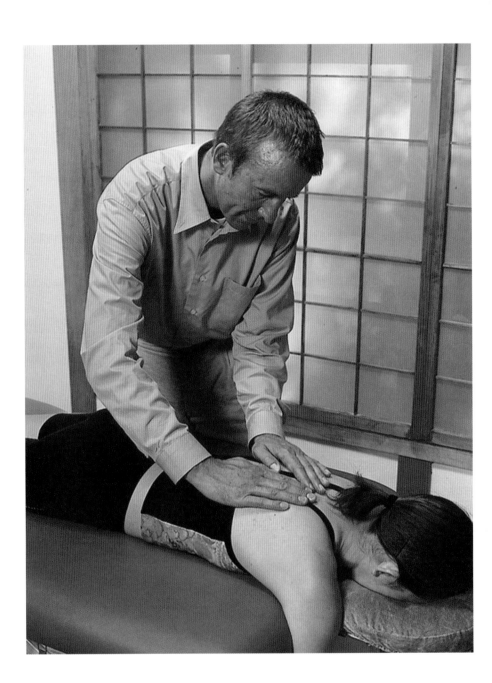

Ketsueki Kokan—The Blood Circulation Technique

Ketsueki Kokan is one of the main Second Degree Reiki Techniques employed by Dr. Hayashi. It can be translated as "blood exchange" but what is meant is "blood circulation". Because the word is complicated, Japanese practitioners usually call the technique *Keko*. Dr. Hayashi suggested using *Keko* at the end of each treatment. It is a rather long process, please practice it diligently. Your clients will love you for it!

1. Push the power symbol into the neck at C 2 (the second cervical vertebra) with the thumb and index finger of your dominant hand.

2. Check where the clients spine is located.

3. With your first and second fingers rub both sides of the spine slowly and carefully two or three times from the first cervical vertebra to the lumbar vertebrae.

4. Once familiar with the client's spine rub it vigorously 20 times.

5. Push the power symbol into the lumbar area around L3 with the thumb and index finger of your dominant hand.

6. Divide the upper part of the body into five parts. First rub from the spine sideways to the shoulders and down to the upper arms four or five times.

7. Second rub from behind the heart down to the sides four or five times.

8. Third rub from the spine behind the solar plexus down to the lower ribs four or five times.

9. Fourth rub from the lower back to the sides four or five times.

10. Fifth, rub from the buttocks to the hips four or five times.

11. Now rub ten times across the small of the back with the palm of your dominant hand while steadying the client with the other hand.

12. Steady the client with one hand and rub with the other on the outside of his right leg from the hip to the ankles and beyond two or three times.

13. Repeat the same with the client's left leg.

14. Steady the client with one hand and rub with the other on the backside of his right leg from the hip to the ankles and beyond two or three times.

15. Repeat the same with the client's left leg.

16. Steady the client with one hand and rub with the other on the inside of his right leg from the hip to the ankles and beyond two or three times.

17. Repeat the same with the client's left leg.

18. Now push the root of the client's left thigh with your left hand (see photo) while you stretch the leg at the ankle with your right hand.

19. Repeat the same with the client's right leg.

20. To end the treatment, pat the whole backside of the body with the palms of your hands. Begin by patting across the back from the shoulders down behind the ribs to the lower back and the buttocks.

21. Pat on the outside of the client's right leg from the hip all the way down to the outside of the small toe.

22. Repeat the same with the client's left leg.

23. Pat on the backside of the client's right leg from the upper thigh all the way down past the soles of the feet to the tips of the toes.

24. Repeat the same with the client's left leg.

25. Pat on the inside of the client's right leg from the hip all the way down to the outside of the big toe.

26. Repeat the same with the client's left leg.

The technique is completed.

After completing this treatment make sure the client has fifteen minutes to come back to the real world.

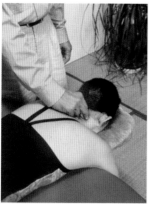

Push the power symbol into the neck at C 2 with thumb and index finger

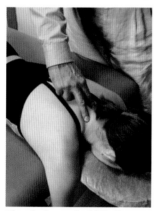

Place index and middle finger on the spine next to C7

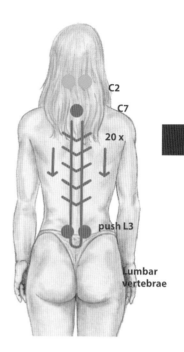

C2
C7
20 x
push L3
Lumbar vertebrae

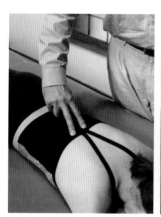

Stroke down alongside the spine

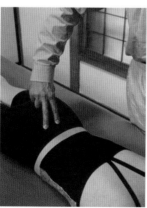

until above the sacrum, L 3-5, twenty times

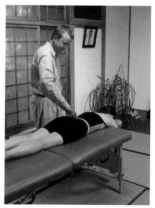

Push power symbol into lumbar area, around L3

53

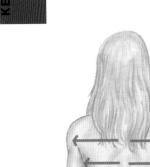

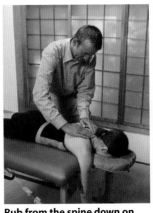

Rub from the spine down on both sides to the shoulders

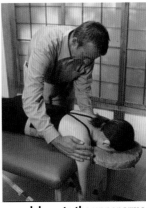

... and down to the upper arms

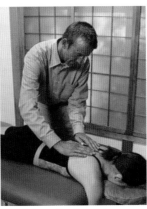

... rub from the heart down

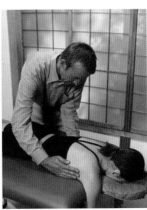

... to the sides of the body

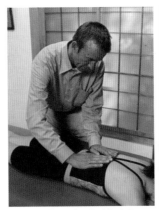

... from the spine behind the ribs

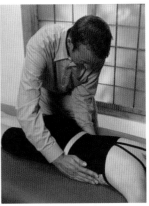

... down to the sides

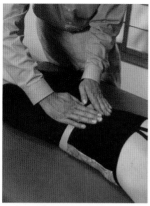
... from the lower back

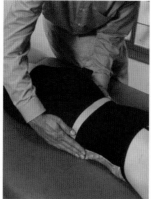
... to the sides

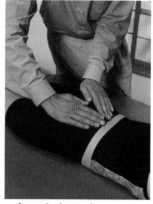
... from the buttocks

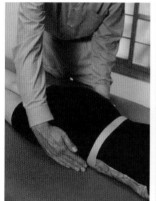
... past the hips to the sides

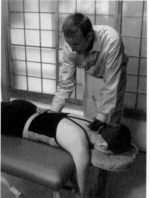
Rub across the small of the back, steady the client with one hand and rub with the other

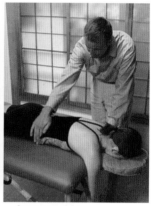
... from one side

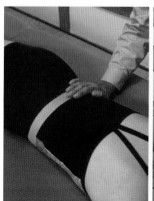
... to the other, 10 times

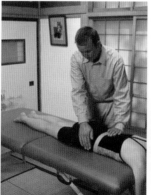
Steady client with one hand and rub with the other on the outside of the leg from hip

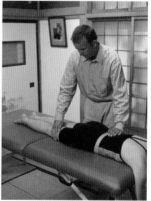
... past the knee

55

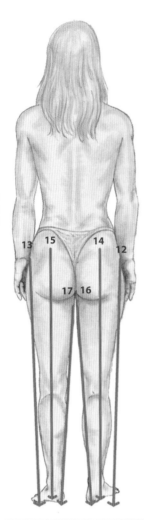

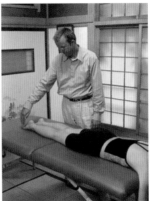

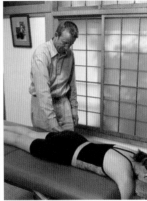

... past the ankle, 2 or three times

Repeat on the other side, from the upper thigh

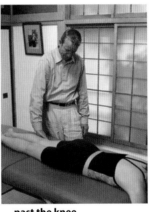

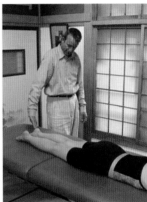

... past the knee

... past the ankle, 2 or three times

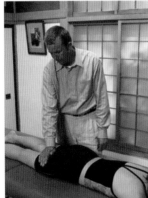

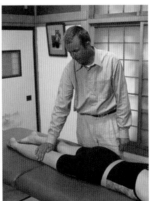

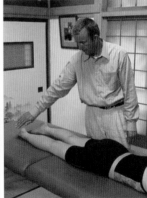

Repeat on the top from the upper thigh

... past the knee

... past the ankle

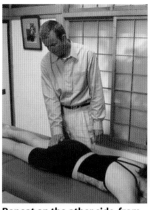
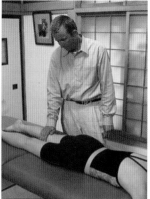
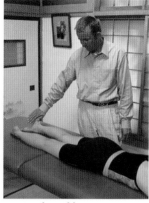

Repeat on the other side, from the upper thigh

... past the knee

... past the ankle

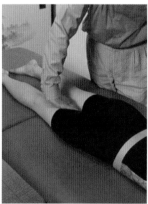
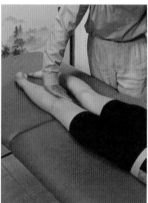
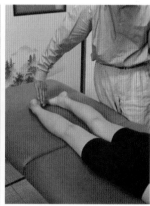

Repeat on the inside of the leg, from the upper thigh

... past the knee

... past the ankle

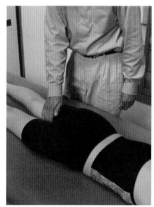
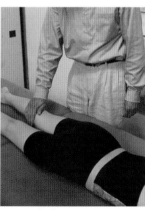
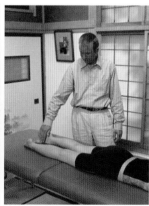

Repeat on the other side on the inside of the leg, from the upper thigh

... past the knee

... past the ankle

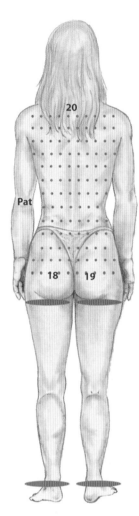

20

Pat

18° 19°

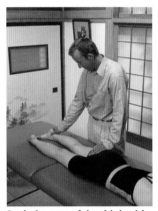

Push the root of the thigh with left hand, while you stretch the ankle with the other hand

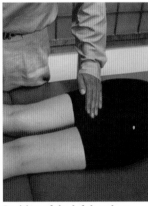

Position of the left hand, on root of thigh

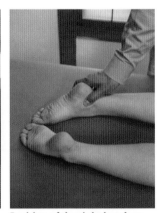

Position of the right hand, on ankle

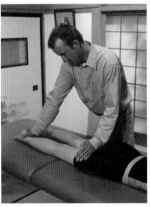

Repeat on the other side

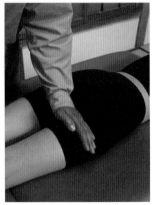

Position of the left hand, on root of thigh

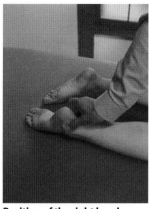

Position of the right hand, on ankle

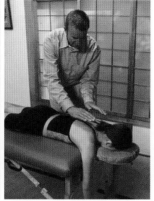

Pat across the back, from the shoulders

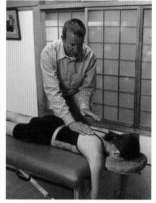

... down behind the ribs

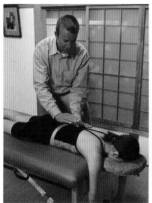

... to the lower back

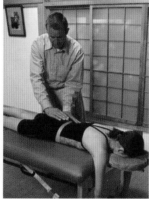

... and the buttocks

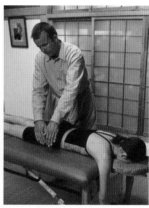

Pat on the side of the leg from the hip

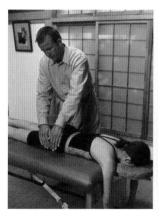

... from the hip down

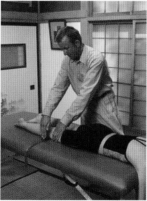

... past the knee

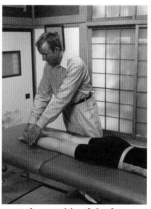

... to the outside of the foot (little toe)

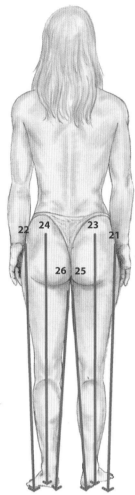

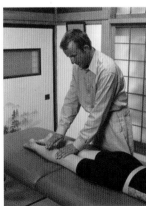

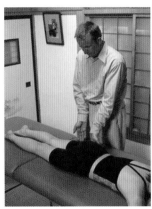

Repeat on the other side, pat from the hip

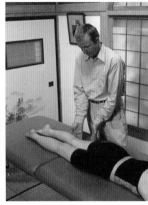

... past the knee

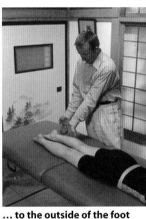

... to the outside of the foot (little toe)

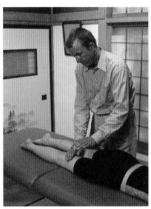

Pat on top of leg from the upper thigh

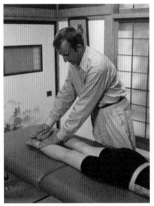

... past the knee

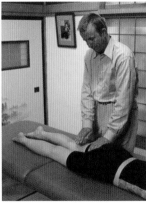

... to the sole of the foot

Repeat on the other side, from the upper thigh

60

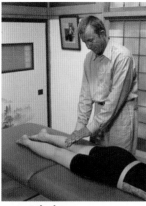
... past the knee

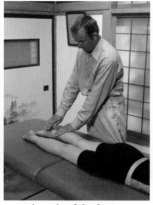
... to the sole of the foot

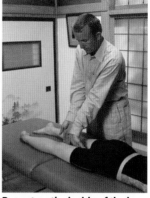
Repeat on the inside of the leg, from the upper thigh

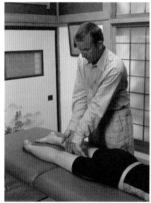
... past the knee and the inside of the foot

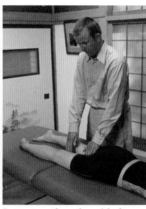
Repeat on the other side from the upper thigh

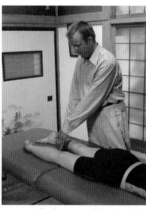
... past the knee and the inside of the foot.

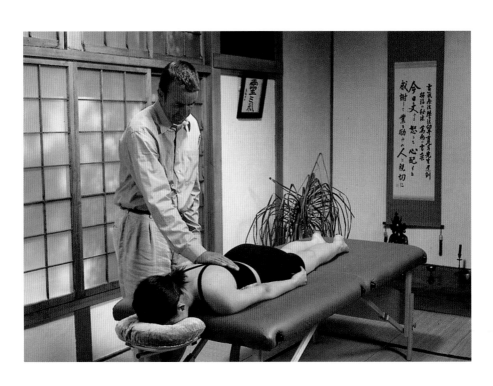

Chapter 5

Ryoho Shishin—The Healing Plan

Healing Techniques as Given by Dr. Chujiro Hayashi

Both Dr. Usui and Dr. Hayashi gave their students handbooks depicting certain positions as well as a copy of the Meiji Emperor's poems. Dr. Hayashi also gave his students Japanese fans with the Reiki Principles written upon them.

The material presented below has been used in Japan for seventy years and was known to Western Reiki practitioners during Hawayo Takata's day. The Japanese original was published in a booklet that is known to have been given to a few members of the Reiki Alliance.

Dr. Hayashi's handbook differs a little from that of his teacher. Since Dr. Hayashi was a physician we find many medical words, the most important of which I have translated or described in modern English. Tadao and I decided to add photographs to the treatment plan to make them easily understood. Most of all we are trying to give you an incentive to use them.

Please be aware of the fact that Ryoho Shishin healing techniques date from the beginning of last century and consider this while reading about the diseases and the accompanying instructions.

If you study this information given to us by Dr. Hayashi you will see clearly how the standard Western Reiki hand positions were later developed.

Part 1:

Head in general

Include the head positions when treating any disease

1. Head:

Brain diseases, headache

1. Forehead, 2. Temples, 3. Back of the head and the tendons in the back of the neck, 4. Top of the head

[Note: Include the head positions as part of the treatment for any disease. For headaches thoroughly treat the area that hurts.]

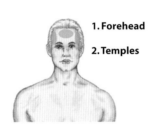

1. Forehead

2. Temples

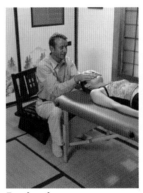

Forehead

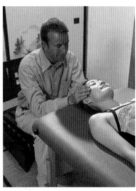

Temples

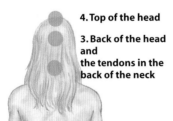

4. Top of the head

3. Back of the head and
the tendons in the
back of the neck

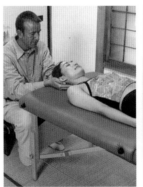

Back of the head

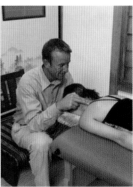

Tendons of the neck

2. Eyes:

All kinds of eye diseases: conjunctivitis, trachoma (infection of the conjunctiva and cornea that may lead to blindness), leucoma, nearsightedness, trichiasis, ptosis, cataract, glaucoma (disorders that lead to atrophy of the optic nerve), etc.
1. Eye balls, 2. Inside corners of eyes, 3. Outside corners of eyes, 4. Back of the head

[Note: Even if only one eye is affected always treat both eyes. You also treat the kidneys, liver, womb, and ovaries.]

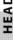
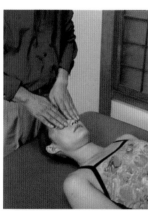

Eye balls

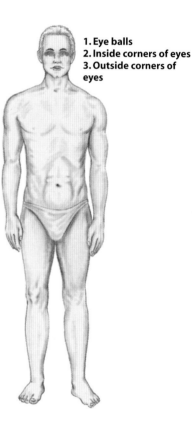

1. Eye balls
2. Inside corners of eyes
3. Outside corners of eyes

Inside corners of eyes

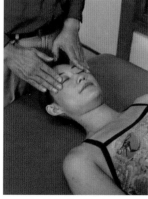

Outside corners of eyes

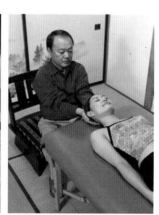

Back of the head

4. Back of the head

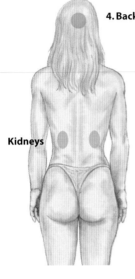

Kidneys

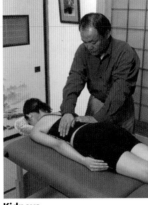

Kidneys

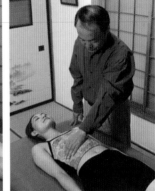

Liver

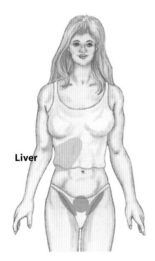

Liver

Womb
Ovaries

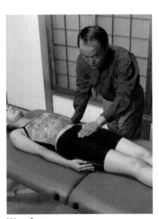

Womb

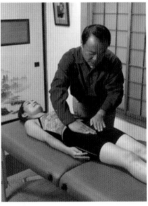

Ovaries

3. Ears:

All kinds of ear diseases, tympanitis, external otitis (outer ear infection), ringing ear, hard of hearing, etc.

1. Auditory canal, 2. The depression just below the ears, 3. The high bone behind the ears, 4. Back of the head

[Note: Even if only one ear has a problem you treat both ears. For diseases that follow influenza, such as tympanitis and parotitis, you must treat bronchi and hilar lymph. Also pay attention to the kidneys, womb, and ovaries.]

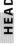

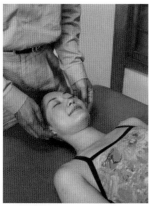

Auditory canal

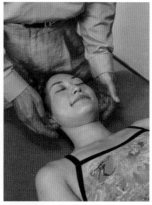

The depression just below the ears

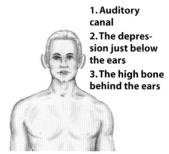

1. Auditory canal
2. The depression just below the ears
3. The high bone behind the ears

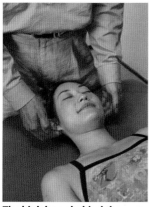

The high bone behind the ears

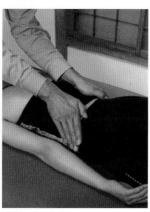

Kidneys

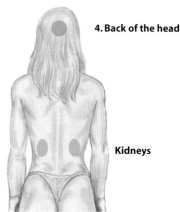

4. Back of the head

Kidneys

67

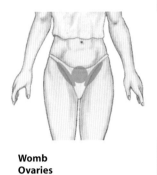

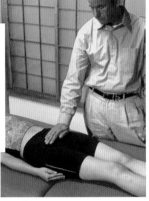

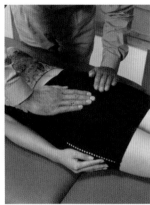

Womb
Ovaries

Womb   **Ovaries**

4. Teeth

In the case of a toothache treat from the outside at the root of the tooth.
Pay attention to the area around the shoulders.

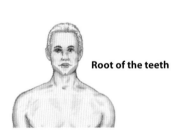

Root of the teeth

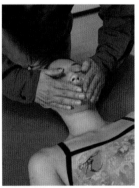

Root of the teeth

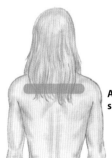

**Area round the
shoulders**

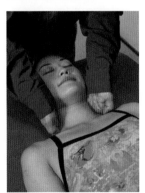

Area round the shoulders

68

5. Oral cavity

Close the mouth and then treat the lips by holding the palms on them.

[Note: see Diseases of Digestive Organs]

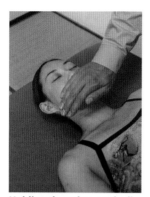

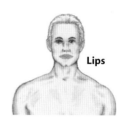

Lips

Holding the palms on the lips

6. Tongue

1. Press on or pinch the diseased part of the tongue
2. Treat the root of the tongue from outside the mouth

[Note: If you find this technique uncomfortable, then press both arches of the feet forward.]

1. Tongue
2. Root of the tongue (outside)

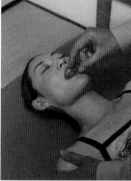

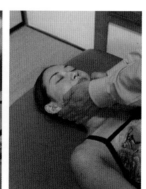

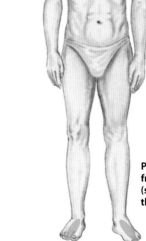

Press on or pinch the diseased part of the tongue

The root o the tongue

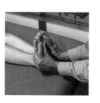

Press both arches of the feet forward

Press forward from the sole (see photo on the left)

Part 2:

Diseases of Digestive Organs

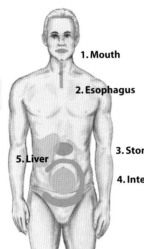

1. Mouth
2. Esophagus
5. Liver
3. Stomach
4. Intestines

1. Stomatitis

(cancer, sores, infection of the inside of the mouth)
1. Mouth, 2. Esophagus, 3. Stomach, 4. Intestines,
5. Liver

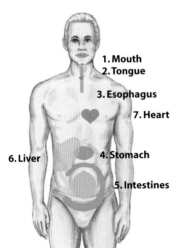

1. Mouth
2. Tongue
3. Esophagus
7. Heart
6. Liver
4. Stomach
5. Intestines

2. Thrush

(Candidiasis, an oral yeast infection, a strand of Candida)
1. Mouth, 2. Tongue, 3. Esophagus, 4. Stomach, 5. Intestines, 6. Liver, 7. Heart, 8. Kidneys

[Note: To heal the tongue, also treat the arches of the feet.]

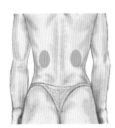

8. Kidneys

Press both arches of the feet forward

70

3. Saliva

Excess salivating, Xerostomia (chronic dryness of the mouth), Sialolithiasis (calcific stones in the ducts of the salivary glands), Parotitis (bacterial infection of the oral cavity often caused by reduced salivary flow. Mumps is one of those infections.)

1. Mouth, 2. Root of the tongue, 3. Stomach, 4. Intestines, 5. Head

5. Head

1. Mouth
2. Root of the tongue

3. Stomach

4. Intestines

4. Esophagus diseases:

Stricture of the esophagus, dilation of the esophagus, esophagi's (infection of esophagus)

1. Esophagus, 2. Cardia (solar plexus), 3. Stomach, 4. Intestines, 5. Liver, 6. Pancreas, 7. Kidneys, 8. Ketsueki Kokan* (blood circulation technique)

[Note: the prognosis for esophagus cancer is most likely not very good.]

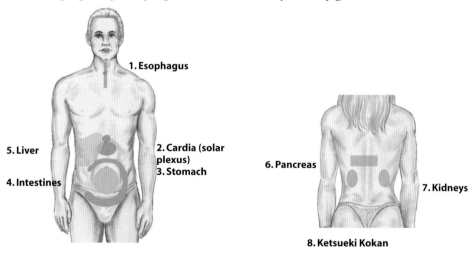

1. Esophagus

5. Liver

2. Cardia (solar plexus)
3. Stomach

4. Intestines

6. Pancreas

7. Kidneys

8. Ketsueki Kokan

---

* The "Ketsueki Kokan, blood circulation technique" is often employed to heal the following diseases. A detailed explanation can be found on pages 51 to 61.

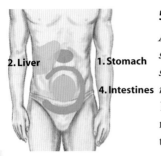

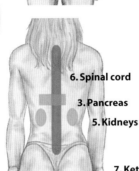

5. Stomach diseases:

Acute and chronic gastritis (inflammation of the stomach), gastric atony, gastric dilation, gastric ulcer, stomach cancer, gastroptosis, neurologic stomach ache, neurologic dyspepsia, (indigestion) gastrospasm

1. Stomach, 2.Liver, 3. Pancreas, 4. Intestines, 5. Kidneys, 6. Spinal cord, 7. Ketsueki Kokan (blood circulation technique)

[Note: If a cancer is obvious the prognosis is most likely not very good.]

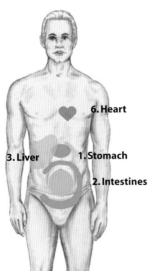

6. Intestinal diseases:

Intestinal catarrh, constipation, appendicitis, vermiform process, ileus (intestinal thrombosis), invagination, intestinal volvulus (intestinal obstruction), intestinal bleeding, diarrhea

1. Stomach, 2. Intestines, 3. Liver, 4. Pancreas, 5. Kidneys, 6. Heart, 7. Ketsueki Kokan (blood circulation technique), 8. Lumbar vertebrae, 9. Sacrum

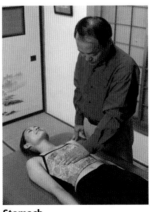

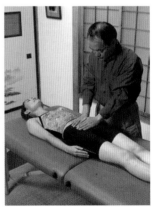

Stomach   Intestines

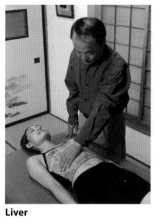
Liver

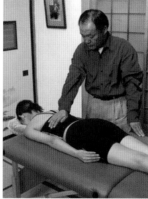
Pancreas

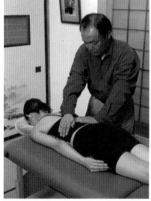
Kidneys

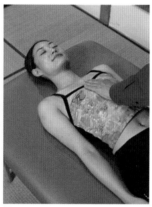
Heart

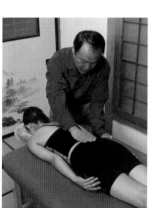
Lumbar vertebrae

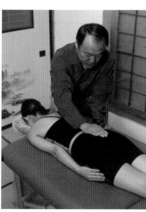
Sacrum

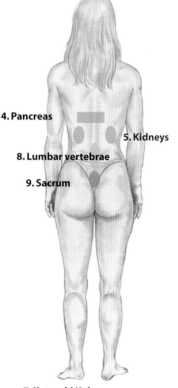

4. Pancreas

5. Kidneys

8. Lumbar vertebrae

9. Sacrum

7. Ketsueki Kokan

73

7. Liver diseases:

Liver congestion, liver hyperemia (excess blood in the liver), abscess, sclerosis, hypertrophy (increase in cell size), atrophy (decrease in function and size of a cell or an organ), jaundice, gallstone, etc.

1. Liver, 2. Pancreas, 3. Stomach, 4. Intestines, 5. Heart, 6. Kidneys, 7. Ketsueki Kokan (blood circulation technique)

[Note: A few days after the treatment the gallstones will break into pieces by themselves and will be eliminated from the body. The prognosis for liver cancer is most likely not very good.]

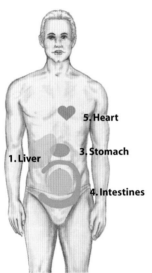

5. Heart

3. Stomach

1. Liver

4. Intestines

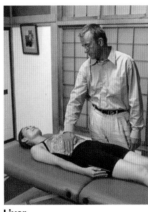

Liver

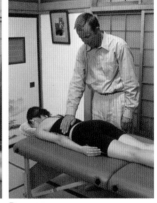

Pancreas

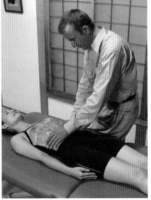

Stomach

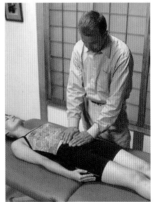

Intestines

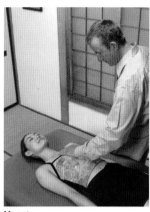

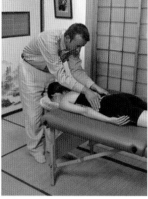

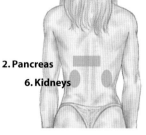

2. Pancreas

6. Kidneys

7. Ketsueki Kokan

Heart

Kidneys

8. Pancreatic diseases:

Liver cyst, ptosis, hypertrophy, etc.

1. Pancreas, 2. Liver, 3. Stomach, 4. Intestines, 5. Heart, 6. Kidneys, 7. Ketsueki Kokan (blood circulation technique)

[Note: The prognosis for pancreatic cancer is most likely not very good.]

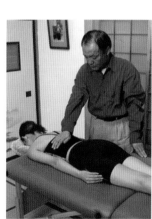

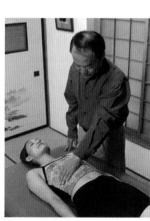

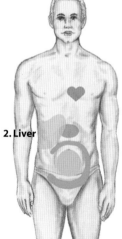

5. Heart

2. Liver

3. Stomach

4. Intestines

Pancreas

Liver

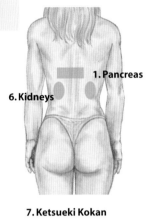

1. Pancreas

6. Kidneys

7. Ketsueki Kokan

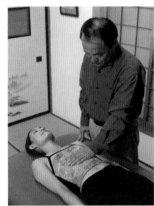

Stomach

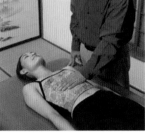

Intestines

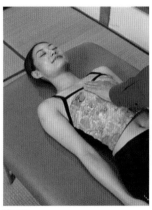

Heart

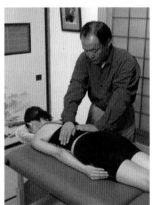

Kidneys

9. Peritoneum diseases, in general

1. Liver, 2. Pancreas, 3. Stomach, 4. Intestines, 5. Peritoneum area, 6. Bladder, 7. Heart, 8. Kidneys, 9. Ketsueki Kokan (blood circulation technique)

[Note: If the patient suffers from tuberculosis as well treat the lungs.]

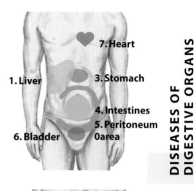

7. Heart
1. Liver
3. Stomach
4. Intestines
5. Peritoneum
6. Bladder 0area

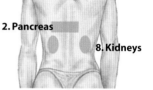

2. Pancreas
8. Kidneys

9. Ketsueki Kokan

10. Anal diseases:

Hemorrhoid, inflammation of anus area, open sores of anus area, bleeding piles, anal fistula, prolapse of the anus

1. The affected part of anus, 2. Coccyges (tailbone), 3. Stomach, 4. Intestines

[Note: When treating anal fistula proceed with the same treatment as for intestinal and pulmonary tuberculosis.]

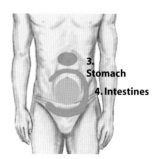

2. Coccyges (tailbone)
1. The affected part of anus

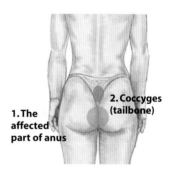

3. Stomach
4. Intestines

Part 3:

Respiratory Diseases

1. Nasal diseases:

Acute and chronic nasal catarrh, hypertrophic and atrophic nasal catarrh

1. Nose, 2. Pharynx, 3. Bronchi (in the lung area)

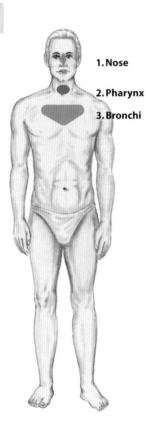

1. Nose

2. Pharynx

3. Bronchi

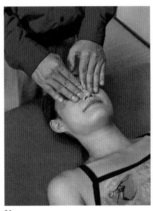

Nose

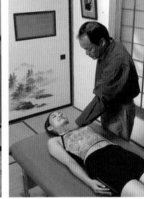

Pharynx

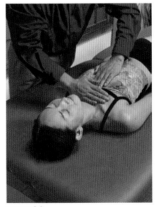

Bronchi

2. Maxillary empyema
(Pleurisy with formation of pus)

1. Nose, 2. Depression of upper forehead, 3. Chest, 4. Pharynx (upper throat), 5. Kidneys, 6. Stomach, 7. Intestines, 8. Ketsueki Kokan (blood circulation technique)

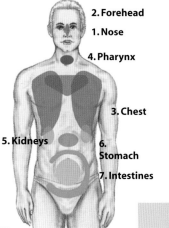

3. Epistaxis (nosebleed)

1. Nasal bones, 2. Back of the head

[Note: If menstruation is late or irregular and nosebleed occurs, treat the womb and ovaries.]

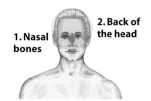

4. Pharyngitis (sore throat) and tonsillitis
(infection of the tonsils)

1. Pharynx, 2. Tonsil area, 3. Bronchi, 4. Kidneys, 5. Lungs, 6. Stomach, 7. Intestines, 8. Head

[Note: For tonsillitis, treat the kidneys well.]

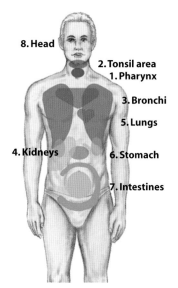

79

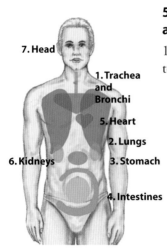

7. Head

1. Trachea and Bronchi

5. Heart

2. Lungs

6. Kidneys

3. Stomach

4. Intestines

5. Tracheitis (infection of the trachea, often as a result of flu) and bronchitis

1. Trachea and bronchi, 2. Lungs, 3. Stomach, 4. Intestines, 5. Heart, 6. Kidneys, 7. Head

6. Pneumonia:

1. Lungs, 2. Bronchi, 3. Heart, 4. Liver, 5. Pancreas, 6. Stomach 7. Intestines, 8. Kidneys, 9. Ketsueki Kokan (blood circulation technique)

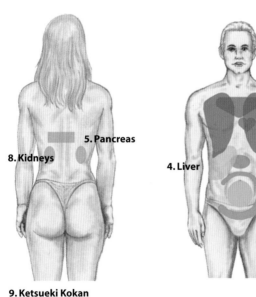

5. Pancreas

8. Kidneys

9. Ketsueki Kokan

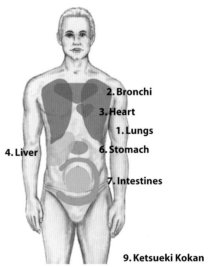

2. Bronchi

3. Heart

1. Lungs

4. Liver

6. Stomach

7. Intestines

9. Ketsueki Kokan

7. Asthma:

Chronic and acute asthma

1. Bronchi, 2. Lungs, 3. Liver, 4. Pancreas, 5. Diaphragm, 6. Stomach, 7. Intestines, 8. Kidneys, 9. Head, 10. Nose, 11. Heart

[Note: During an acute attack treat your patient sitting up.]

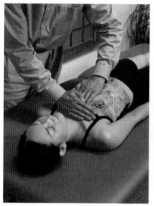

Bronchi

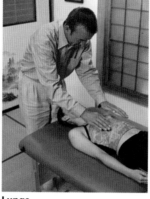

Lungs

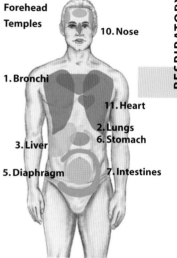

Forehead
Temples
10. Nose
1. Bronchi
11. Heart
2. Lungs
3. Liver
6. Stomach
5. Diaphragm
7. Intestines

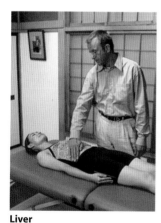

Liver

Pancreas

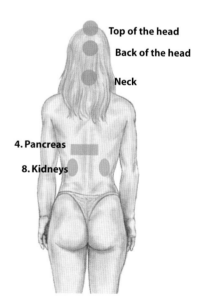

Top of the head
Back of the head
Neck
4. Pancreas
8. Kidneys

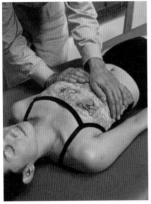

Diaphragm

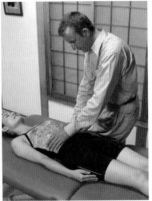

Stomach

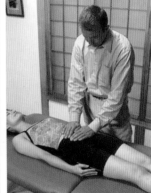

Intestines

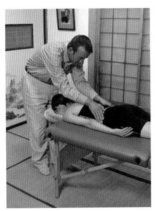

Kidneys

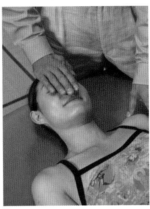

Nose

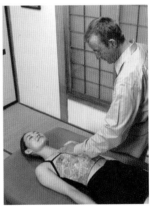

Heart

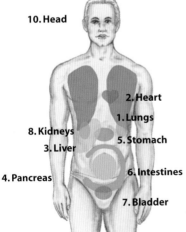

10. Head
2. Heart
1. Lungs
8. Kidneys
5. Stomach
3. Liver
4. Pancreas
6. Intestines
7. Bladder
9. Spinal cord

8. Lung diseases:

Pulmonary edema (excess fluid in the lungs), abscess, pulmonary tuberculosis, emphysema of lungs (enlargement of the air spaces distal to the terminal bronchioles)

1. Lung area, 2. Heart, 3. Liver, 4. Pancreas, 5. Stomach, 6. Intestines, 7. Bladder, 8. Kidneys, 9. Spinal cord, 10. Head

[Note: In a female patient regardless of her age always treat the womb and the ovaries. "Ketsueki Kokan" is effective, but do not do it with very weak and very sick patients.]

9. Pleurisy (infection of the pleura):

Both dry and moist
1. Chest area in general, 2. Heart, 3. Liver, 4. Pancreas,
5. Stomach, 6. Intestines, 7. Kidneys, 8. Ketsueki
Kokan (blood circulation technique)

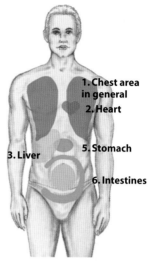

1. Chest area in general
2. Heart
3. Liver
5. Stomach
6. Intestines

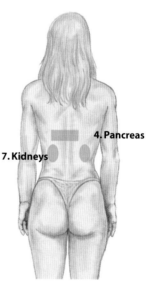

4. Pancreas
7. Kidneys

8. Ketsueki Kokan

Part 4

Cardiovascular Diseases

1. Heart diseases:

Endocarditis (infection of the heart valves), endocardium diseases, various symptoms of pericardium, various symptoms of the heart itself, palpitation, angina pectoris, etc.

1. Heart, 2. Liver, 3. Stomach, 4. Intestines, 5. Pancreas, 6. Kidneys, 7. Spinal cord, 8. Ketsueki Kokan (blood circulation technique)

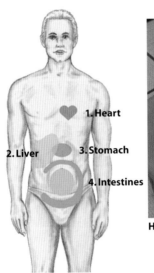

1. Heart
2. Liver
3. Stomach
4. Intestines

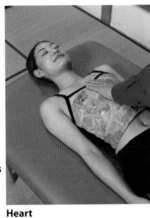

Heart

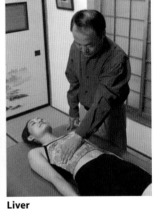

Liver

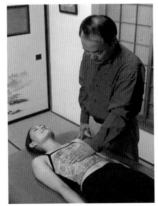

Stomach

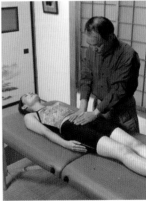

Intestines

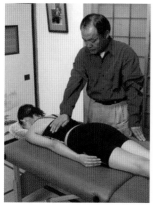

Pancreas

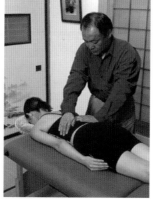

Kidneys

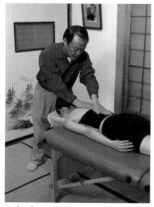

Spinal cord

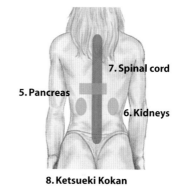

7. Spinal cord

5. Pancreas

6. Kidneys

8. Ketsueki Kokan

2. Arteriosclerosis (arterial calcification)

Aneurysms (dilation of blood vessels), cardiac asthma, etc.,

1. Same as treating heart problems, 2. Bronchi and chest area

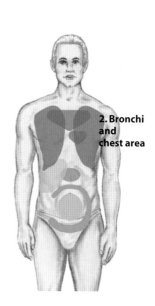

2. Bronchi and chest area

85

Part 5:

Urinary Organ Diseases

1. Kidney diseases:

Kidney congestion, nephrogenic anemia (reduction of hemoglobin count), atrophy, sclerosis, hypertrophy, abscess, wandering kidney, pyelitis (cystic lesions of the urinary tract), kidney stone, uremia (chronically elevated level of blood urea nitrogen), filariasis (inflammation due to filarial worms)

1. Kidneys, 2. Liver, 3. Pancreas, 4. Heart, 5. Stomach, 6. Intestines, 7. Bladder, 8. Head, 9. Ketsueki Kokan (blood circulation technique)

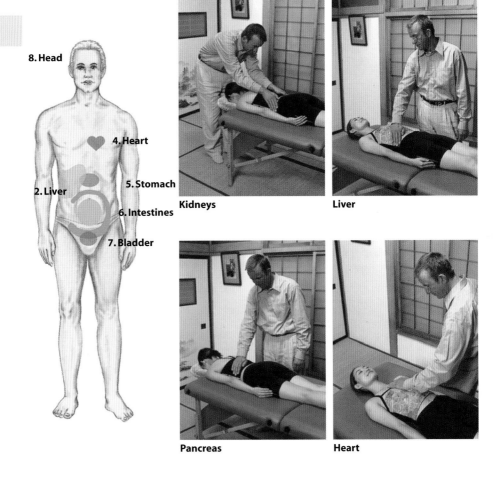

8. Head

4. Heart

2. Liver

5. Stomach

6. Intestines

7. Bladder

Kidneys

Liver

Pancreas

Heart

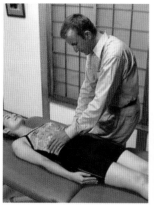

Stomach

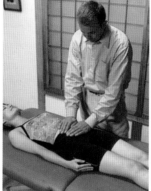

Intestines

3. Pancreas

1. Kidneys

9. Ketsueki Kokan

Bladder

2. Cystitis (inflammation of the bladder): urinary retention, uremia, urgency, pain when urinating.

1. Kidneys, 2. Bladder, 3. Urethra, 4. Prostate gland, 5. Womb, 6. Same as treating kidney diseases

3. Enuresis (bed wetting)

1. Bladder, 2. Intestines, 3. Stomach, 4. Kidneys, 5. Spinal cord, 6. Head, 7. Ketsueki Kokan (blood circulation technique)

Part 6:

Neurological Diseases

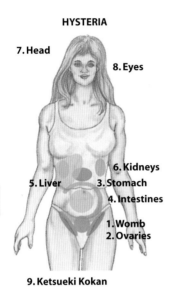

HYSTERIA

7. Head

8. Eyes

6. Kidneys
5. Liver
3. Stomach
4. Intestines
1. Womb
2. Ovaries

9. Ketsueki Kokan

1. Cerebral anemia, cerebral hyperemia (vascular congestion in the brain)

1. Head, 2. Heart

2. Hysteria

1. Womb, 2. Ovaries, 3. Stomach, 4. Intestines, 5. Liver, 6. Kidneys, 7. Head, 8. Eyes, 9. Ketsueki Kokan (blood circulation technique)

3. Nervous breakdown, insomnia (sleeplessness)

1. Stomach, 2. Intestines, 3. Liver, 4. Pancreas, 5. Kidneys, 6. Eyes, 7. Head, 8. Ketsueki Kokan (blood circulation technique)

[Note: Do it very gently in case of maxillary empyema.]

4. Meningitis

1. Head area: treat mainly the back of the head and the tendons in the back of the neck.

[Note: Mainly treat the head in order to heal the root cause of the disease. Treat the nose, the forehead, and the area of inflammation of the head. Also in order to heal diseases in remote organs such as gastritis and pneumonia caused by erysipelas. Same treatment as for tuberculosis.]

5. Epidemic cerebrospinal meningitis

1. Spinal cord, 2. Back of the head and the tendons in the back of the neck, 3. Heart, 4. Stomach, 5. Intestines, 6. Liver, 7. Kidneys, 8. Bladder

[Note: Mainly treat the spinal cord, the back of the head, and the tendons in the back of the neck.]

6. Myelitis (inflammation of the spinal cord)

1. Spinal cord in general, 2. Stomach, 3. Intestines, 4. Liver, 5. Bladder, 6. Kidneys, 7. Head, 8. Ketsueki Kokan (blood circulation technique)

7. Cerebral hemorrhage:

Intracerebral bleeding, cerebral thrombosis, etc.
1. Head, 2. Heart, 3. Kidneys, 4. Stomach, 5. Intestines, 6. Liver, 7. Spinal cord, 8. Paralyzed area

8. Polio

1. Spinal cord, 2. Stomach, 3. Intestines, 4. Kidneys, 5. Sacrum, 6. Paralyzed area, 7. Head, 8. Ketsueki Kokan (blood circulation technique)

9. Neuralgia (nerve pain), palsy, neural spasticity, migraine

1. Affected area, 2. Liver, 3. Pancreas, 4. Stomach, 5. Intestines, 6. Kidneys, 7. Head, 8. Spinal cord, 9. Ketsueki Kokan (blood circulation technique)

[Note: Pay attention to the womb and the ovaries.]

10. Beriberi

1. Stomach, 2. Intestines, 3. Heart, 4. Liver, 5. Pancreas, 6. Kidneys, 7. Paralyzed or edematous area, 8. Ketsueki Kokan (blood circulation technique)

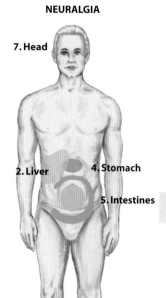

7. Head
2. Liver
4. Stomach
5. Intestines

9. Ketsueki Kokan

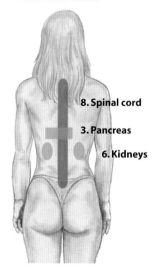

8. Spinal cord
3. Pancreas
6. Kidneys

POISONING

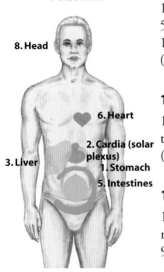

8. Head

6. Heart

2. Cardia (solar plexus)

3. Liver

1. Stomach

5. Intestines

4. Pancreas

7. Kidneys

9. Ketsueki Kokan

11. Basedow's Disease (Graves' disease, auto-immune disease often leading to hyperthyroidism)

1. Womb, 2. Ovaries, 3. Stomach, 4. Intestines, 5. Liver, 6. Pancreas, 7. Heart, 8. Thyroid, 9. Eyes, 10. Kidneys, 11. Spinal cord, 12. Ketsueki Kokan (blood circulation technique)

12. Epilepsy

1. Liver, 2. Pancreas, 3. Head, 4. Stomach, 5. Intestines, 6. Kidneys, 7. Spinal cord, 8. Ketsueki Kokan (blood circulation technique)

13. Convulsion

1. Liver, 2. Stomach, 3. Intestines, 4. Kidneys, 5. Spinal cord, 6. Shoulders, 7. Arms, 8. Elbow joint area, 9. Wrist, 10. Head

14. Chorea (Huntington's disease, involuntary movements of all body parts etc.)

1. Liver, 2. Stomach, 3. Intestines, 4. Kidneys, 5. Spinal cord, 6. Spastic area at the legs, feet, arms and hands, 7. Head, 8. Ketsueki Kokan (blood circulation technique)

15. Sea sickness

1. Stomach, 2. Solar Plexus, 3. Head

16. Poisoning, food poisoning, addictions

1. Stomach, 2. Solar Plexus, 3. Liver, 4. Pancreas, 5. Intestines, 6. Heart, 7. Kidneys, 8. Head, 9. Ketsueki Kokan (blood circulation technique)

Part 7:

Infectious Diseases

1. Typhoid fever, paratyphoid fever

1. Liver, 2. Pancreas (spleen), 3. Stomach, 4. Intestines, 5. Heart, 6. Kidneys, 7. Spinal cord, 8. Head

2. Dysentery:

Cholera, children's dysentery and others
1. Stomach, 2. Intestines, 3. Liver, 4. Pancreas, 5. Kidneys, 6. Heart, 7. Head, 8. Ketsueki Kokan (blood circulation technique)

3. Measles

1. Pharynx, 2. Trachea, 3. Bronchi, 4. Stomach, 5. Intestines, 6. Heart, 7. Kidneys, 8. Spinal cord, 9. Head

4. Scarlatina (scarlet fever)

1. Pharynx, 2. Chest, 3. Kidneys, 4. Stomach, 5. Intestines, 6. Bladder, 7. Head, 8. Ketsueki Kokan (blood circulation technique)

5. Varicella (chicken pox) and herpes zoster (shingles)

1. Stomach, 2. Intestines, 3. Kidneys, 4. Ketsueki Kokan, blood circulation technique, 5. Affected area, 6. Head

MEASLES

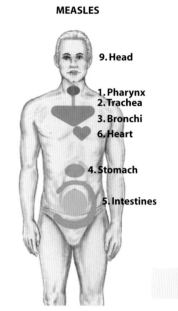

9. Head
1. Pharynx
2. Trachea
3. Bronchi
6. Heart
4. Stomach
5. Intestines

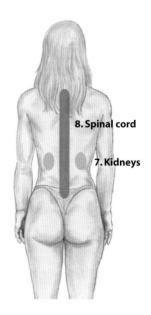

8. Spinal cord
7. Kidneys

INFECTIOUS DISEASES

6. Influenza Virus (flu)

1. Nose, 2. Pharynx, 3. Trachea, 4. Bronchi, 5. Lungs, 6. Liver, 7. Pancreas, 8. Stomach, 9. Intestines, 10. Kidneys, 11. Head area, 12. Ketsueki Kokan (blood circulation technique)

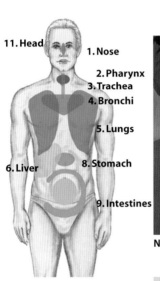

11. Head
1. Nose
2. Pharynx
3. Trachea
4. Bronchi
5. Lungs
8. Stomach
6. Liver
9. Intestines

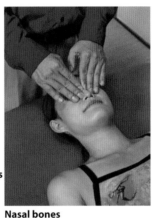

Nasal bones

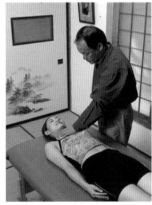

Pharynx

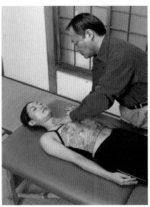

Trachea

Bronchi

92

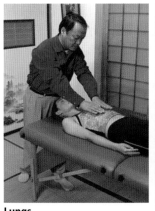

Lungs

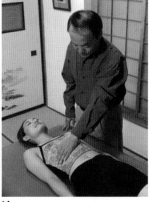

Liver

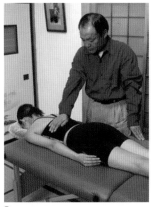

Pancreas

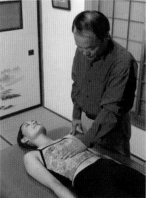

Stomach

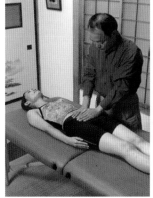

Intestines

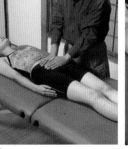

Kidneys

11. Head area

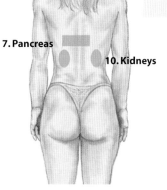
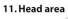

7. Pancreas

10. Kidneys

12. Ketsueki Kokan

93

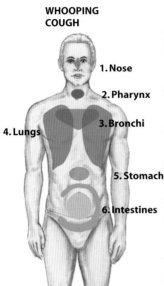

WHOOPING COUGH

1. Nose
2. Pharynx
3. Bronchi
4. Lungs
5. Stomach
6. Intestines

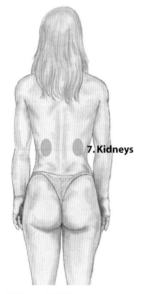

7. Kidneys

8. Ketsueki Kokan

7. Whooping cough, pertusis (upper respiratory tract infection)

1. Nose, 2. Pharynx, 3. Bronchi, 4. Apex of the lungs, 5. Stomach, 6. Intestines, 7. Kidneys, 8. Ketsueki Kokan (blood circulation technique)

8. Diphtheria

1. Pharynx, 2. Trachea, 3. Nose, 4. Lungs, 5. Heart, 6. Liver, 7. Stomach, 8. Intestines, 9. Kidneys, 10. Head, 11. Ketsueki Kokan (blood circulation technique)

9. Weil's Disease (acute infectious disease caused by leptospiral bacteria)

1. Liver, 2. Pancreas (spleen), 3. Stomach, 4. Intestines, 5. Bladder, 6. Kidneys, 7. Spinal cord, 8. Head, 9. Ketsueki Kokan (blood circulation technique)

10. Malaria

1. Pancreas (spleen), 2. Liver, 3. Heart, 4. Stomach, 5. Intestines, 6. Kidneys, 7. Spinal cord, 8. Ketsueki Kokan (blood circulation technique)

11. Tetanus (lockjaw)

1. Jawbone, 2. Back of head, 3. Throat, 4. Lungs, 5. Affected area, 6. Stomach, 7. Intestines, 8. Kidneys, 9. Spinal cord

[Note: In case of puerperal tetanus, treat the womb. In case the child is the first child of the mother, treat the navel as well.]

12. Articular rheumatism, muscular rheumatism

1. Affected area, 2. Heart, 3. Chest, 4. Liver, 5. Pancreas, 6. Stomach, 7. Intestines, 8. Kidneys, 9. Spinal cord, 10. Head

13. Rabies

1. Affected area, 2. Heart, 3. Liver, 4. Kidneys, 5. Stomach, 6. Intestines, 7. Spinal cord, 8. Pharynx, 9. Head, 10. Ketsueki Kokan (blood circulation technique)

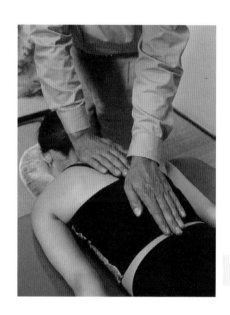

Spinal cord

Part 8:

Diseases of the Whole Body

1. Anemia, leukemia, scorbutus (scurvy)

1. Heart, 2. Liver, 3. Pancreas, 4. Stomach, 5. Intestines, 6. Kidneys, 7. Spinal cord, 8. Ketsueki Kokan (blood circulation technique)

2. Diabetes

1. Liver, 2. Pancreas, 3. Heart, 4. Stomach, 5. Intestines, 6. Bladder, 7. Kidneys, 8. Head, 9. Spinal cord, 10. Ketsueki Kokan (blood circulation technique)

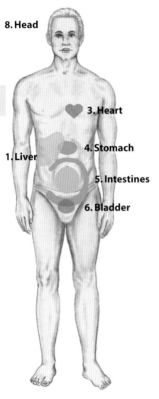

8. Head
3. Heart
4. Stomach
1. Liver
5. Intestines
6. Bladder

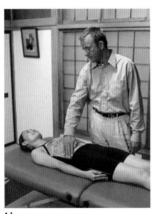

Liver

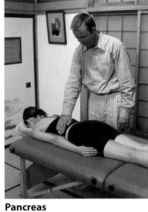

Pancreas

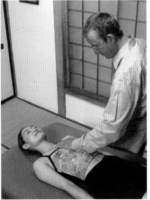

Heart

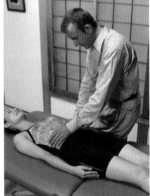

Stomach

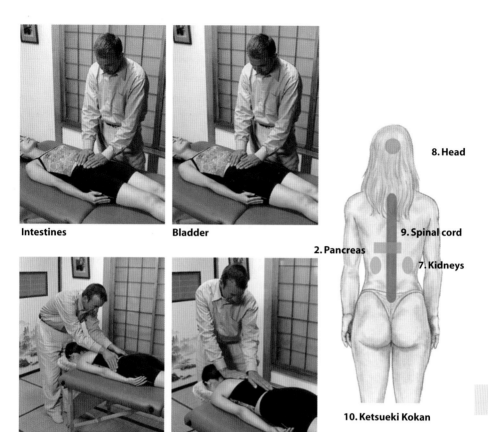

Intestines

Bladder

Kidneys

Spinal cord

8. Head

9. Spinal cord

2. Pancreas

7. Kidneys

10. Ketsueki Kokan

3. Dermatological diseases

1. Stomach, 2. Intestines, 3. Liver, 4. Kidneys, 5. Affected area, 6. Ketsueki Kokan (blood circulation technique)

4. Adiposis (obesity)

The same as diabetes.

5. Scrofula, struma (goiter)

1. Affected area, 2. Stomach, 3. Intestines, 4. Liver, 5. Heart, 6. Chest, 7. Kidneys, 8. Spinal cord, 9. Ketsueki Kokan (blood circulation technique)

Part 9:

Other Diseases and Symptoms

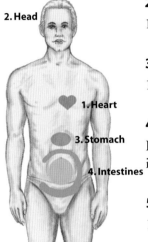

**INFANTILE
CONVULSION**

2. Head

1. Heart

3. Stomach

4. Intestines

1. Infantile convulsion

1. Heart, 2. Head, 3. Stomach, 4. Intestines

2. Child congenital syphilis

1. Affected area, 2. Antidote *(doku kudashi)*

3. Wrong position of fetus

1. Womb

4. Pregnancy

If you treat the womb continually the growth of fetus is healthy.

5. Delivery

1. Sacrum, 2. Lumbar vertebrae

[Note: If you treat these areas the baby will be born smoothly after twelve labor pains. If you keep on treating these areas after the birth the afterbirth will be easy as well.]

6. Death of fetus

If you treat the womb the dead fetus will naturally come out on the same day or the next day.

7. Cessation of mother's milk

If you treat around the breast and mammary gland the mother will soon start having milk.

8. Morning sickness

1. Womb, 2. Stomach, 3. Solar Plexus, 4. Intestines, 5. Kidneys, 6. Head, 7. Spinal cord

9. Erysipelas (streptococcal infection)

1. Affected area, 2. Stomach, 3. Intestines, 4. Liver, 5. Heart, 6. Kidneys, 7. Spinal cord, 8. Ketsueki Kokan (blood circulation technique)

10. Hyperhidrosis

1. Kidneys, 2. Affected area, 3. Ketsueki Kokan (blood circulation technique)

11. Burns

Put one hand one or two inches away from the affected area. When the pain is gone put the hand directly on this area.

12. Cut by a sword (and other cut wounds)

Treat as you press the cut with your thumb or palm to prevent bleeding.

13. Unconsciousness caused by falling, electric shock. etc.

1. *Katsu**, 2. Heart, 3. Head

14. Drowning

1. Help the patient to throw up to expel the water, 2. *Katsu**, 3. Heart, 4. Head

15. Menopause, period pains

1. Womb, 2. Ovaries, 3. Sacrum

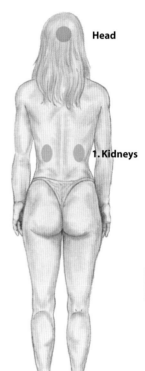

HYPERHIDROSIS

Head

1. Kidneys

3. Ketsueki Kokan

I suggest not to use this technique unless you have been properly instructed in its use.

* *Katsu:* A technique from the martial arts tradition to revive a client. The client lies on his belly and the practitioner places his non-dominant hand on the back of his solar plexus. The dominant hand is then placed on top of the non dominant one. He presses down suddenly and firmly using his own weight and his out breath. As he breathes out and presses down he shouts from his *Dantien* (two or three fingers width below the navel): "Katsu!"

16. Hiccup

1. Diaphragm, 2. Liver, 3. Pancreas, 4. Kidneys, 5. Stomach, 6. Intestines, 7. Spinal cord, 8. Head

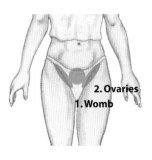

2. Ovaries
1. Womb

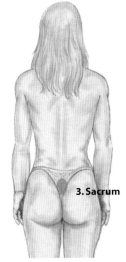

3. Sacrum

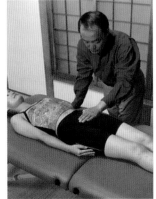

Womb

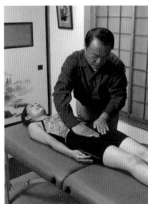

Ovaries

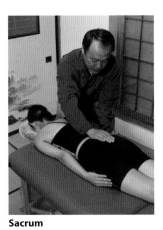

Sacrum

17. Stuttering

1. Pharynx, 2. Head, 3. Singing practice

Practice song number 1:

"Mukou no Koike ni "Dojo" ga sanbiki nyoro-nyoro to" (Three loaches are wiggling in the pond over there.)

100

Practice song number 2:

"Oya ga Kahyo nara ko ga Kahyo. Ko-Kahyo ni Mago-Kahyo" (The parent is Kahyo, the child is Kahyo. Child Kahyo and grandchild Kahyo.)

[Note: Those able to sing these songs can be healed.]

18. Pain at the tip of fingers

1. Affected area

19. Vomiting

1. Stomach, 2. Solar Plexus, 3. Liver, 4. Spinal cord at the back of stomach, 5. Head, 6. Kidneys

20. Splinters

1. Affected area

[Note: When the pain is gone the splinter rises. You pull it out at this moment.]

21. Gonorrhea

1. Urethra, 2. Anal sphincter (Hui-Yin Point), 3. Bladder, 4. Womb

[Note: If it is orchitis (chronic inflammation of the testis) apply your hand lightly on the testicles.]

22. Spasm of pain, stomach cramps

1. Stomach, 2. On the back at the stomach, 3. Liver, 4. Kidneys, 5. Intestines, 6. Head

23. Hernia

As you touch the affected area lightly it will contract by itself. Treat stomach and intestines.

OTHER DISEASES
AND SYMPTOMS

A Final Word

After his awakening on Mount Kurama Dr. Usui set out to convert his satori on the mountain into a tangible reality for his fellow travelers.

The formless manifested as Reiki Ryoho, a dream become reality.

Because of his early death in 1926 a competent student was needed to continue the work. This student was found in Dr. Hayashi who followed the call with utmost devotion even though he was never elected chairperson or official Usui successor of the Usui Reiki Ryoho Gakkai.

Not a single day goes by without the authors' gratitude to Dr. Usui and Dr. Hayashi for what they have given to humankind. This gratitude we would like to extend to you dear reader, for it is only with your help that Reiki can heal the wounds of the world.

Photo Appendix

Hand positions of the Hayashi Reiki-Ryoho Shishin

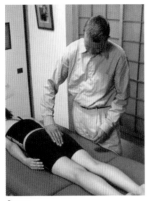

Anus

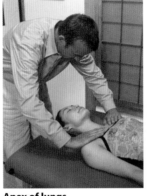

Apex of lungs

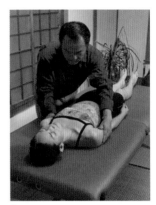

Arms

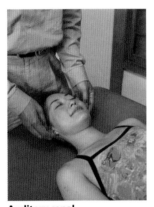

Auditory canal

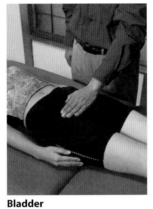

Bladder

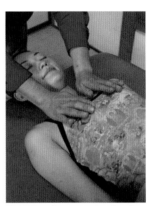

Breast and mammary glands

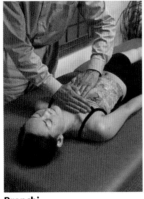

Bronchi

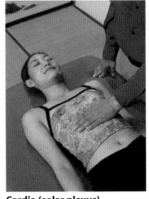

Cardia (solar plexus)

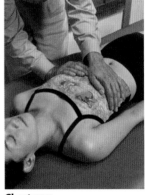

Chest area

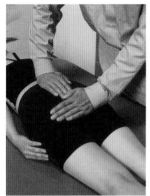

Coccyges (tailbone)

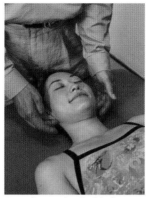

Ears, depression behind

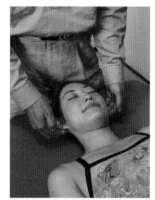

Ears, high bone behind

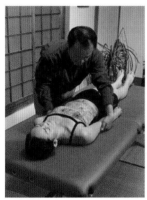

Elbows

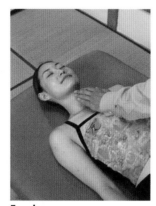

Esophagus

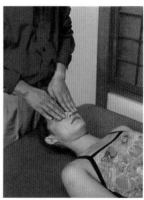

Eye balls

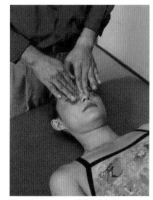

Eyes, corners of (inside)

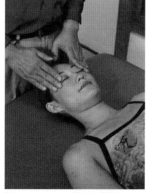

Eyes, corners of (outside)

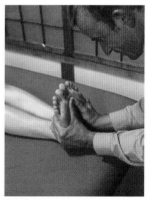

Feet[6]

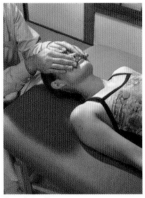

Forehead[1]

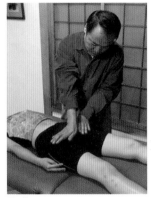

Groin

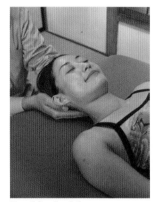

Head, back of the

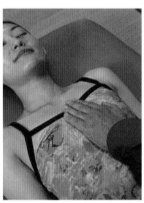

Heart

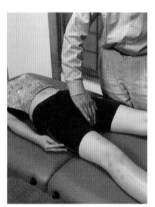

Hui-Yin-Point

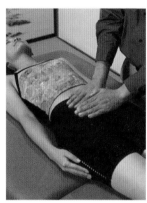

Intestines

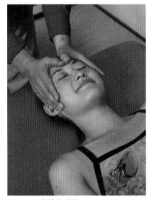

Jaw and Third Eye

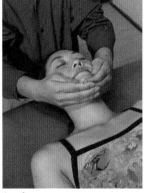

Jaw bone

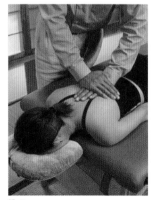

Katsu

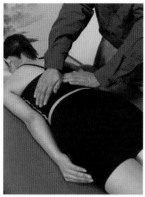

Kidneys

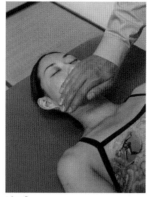

Lips[5]

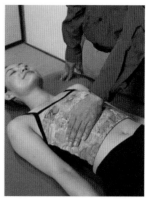

Liver

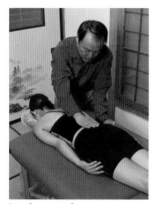

Lumbar vertebrae

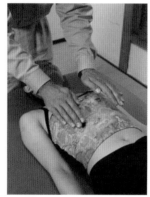

Lungs

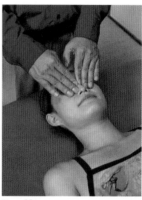

Nasal bones

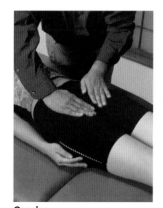

Ovaries

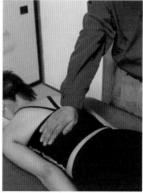

Pancreas

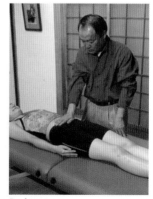

Peritoneum

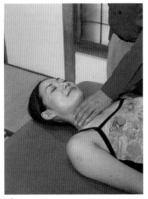

Pharynx

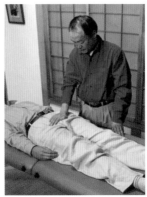

Prostate

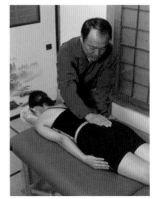

Sacrum

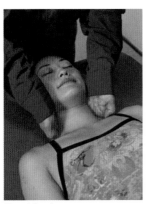

Shoulders[4]

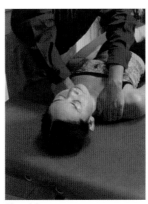

Shoulders

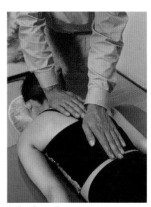

Spinal cord

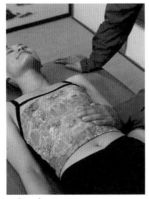

Spleen[2]

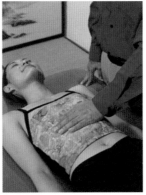

Stomach

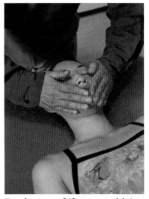

Teeth, root of (from outside)

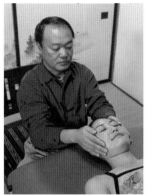
Temples

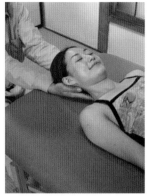
Tendons of the neck

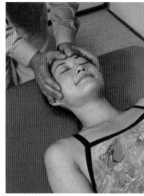
Third Eye

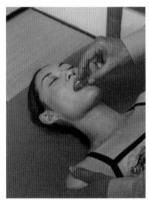
Tongue, press or pinch

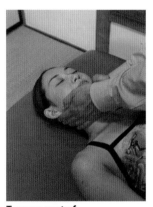
Tongue, root of

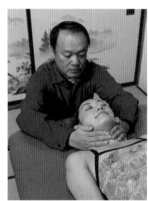
Tonsil area

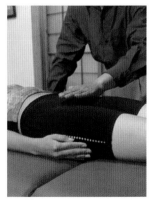
Womb[1]

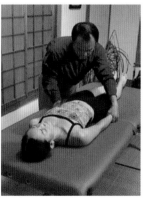
Wrists

1: If you treat the womb, also treat the forehead.

2: The other hand needn't be placed on the head.

3: For treating unconsciousness caused by falling, electric shock, etc.

4: If you treat the teeth, also treat the shoulders.

5: Hold the palms on the lips while the mouth is closed.

6: Press both arches of the feet forward.

The Original Reiki Handbook of Dr. Mikao Usui

by Dr. Mikao Usui and Frank Arjava Petter

Nothing is more authentic than the original Dr. Mikao Usui developed the Reiki System and founded the original "Japanese Usui Reiki Ryoho Gakkai" organization. So what would be more obvious than returning to Dr. Usui's material? This book will show you the original hand positions from Dr. Usui's Reiki handbook.

It has been illustrated with 100 photos to make it easier to understand. The hand positions for a great variety of health complaints have been listed in detail, making it a valuable reference work for anyone who practices Reiki. Now that the original handbook has been translated into English, Dr. Usui's hand positions and healing techniques can be studied directly for the first time. Whether you are an initiate or a master, if you practice Reiki you can expand your knowledge dramatically as you follow in the footsteps of a great healer.

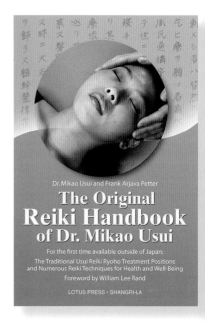

"This information will create a powerful shift in the Reiki community, helping to bring unity at the same time it improves the authenticity of the practice as well as the value it offers. I am sure that all who read this book will benefit in many ways."
— **WILLIAM LEE RAND**
  Author: Reiki for a New Millennium

"A further milestone for the research into the Reiki system—again by Frank Arjava Petter. Reiki friends from all over the world finally receive a detailed description of Usui's original hand positions for the treatment of certain body areas and health disorders."
— **WALTER LÜBECK**
  Author: The Complete Reiki Handbook

The Original
Reiki-Handbook
Dr. Mikao Usui and
Frank Arjava Petter
ISBN: 978-0-9149-5557-3
$14.95 • 80 pp

Available at bookstores and natural food stores nationwide or order your copy directly by sending cost of item plus $2.50 shipping/handling ($.75 s/h for each additional copy ordered at the same time) to:

Lotus Press, PO Box 325, Twin Lakes, WI 53181 USA
toll free order line: 800 824 6396 • office phone: 262 889 856 • office fax: 262 889 2461
email: lotuspress@lotuspress.com • web site: www.lotuspress.com

Lotus Press is the publisher of a wide range of books and software in the field of alternative health, including Ayurveda, Chinese medicine, herbology, aromatherapy, Reiki and energetic healing modalities. Request our free book catalog.

More titles by Frank Arjava Petter

Reiki – The Legacy of Dr. Usui

Rediscover documents on the origins and developements of the Reiki system, as well as new aspects of the Reiki energy

A great deal has been written and said to date about the history of Reiki and his founder. Now Frank Ajarva Petter a Reiki-Master, who lives in Japan, has come across documents that quote Mikao Usui's original words. Questions that his students asked and he answered throw light upon Usui's very personal view of the teachings. Materials meant as the basis for his student's studies round off the entire work. A family tree of the Reiki successors is also included here. In a number of essays, Frank Ajarva Petter also discusses topics related to Reiki and the viewpoints of an independent Reiki teacher.

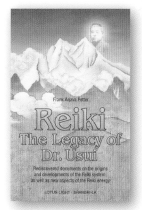

ISBN: 978-0-9149-5556-6
$12.95 • 128 pp

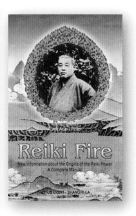

ISBN: 978-0-9149-5550-4
$12.95 • 128 pp

Reiki Fire

New Information about the Origins of the Reiki Power

A Complete Manual

The origin of Reiki has come to be surrounded by many stories and myths. The author, an independent Reiki Master practicing in Japan, immerses it in a new light as he traces Usui-san's path back through time with openness and devotion. He meets Usui's descendants and climbs the holy mountain of his enlightenment.

Reiki, shaped by Shintoism, is a Buddhist expression of Qigong whereby Qigong depicts the teaching of life energy in its original sense. An excellent textbook, fresh and rousing in its spiritual perspective, this is an absolutely practical Reiki guide. The heart, the body, the mind, and esoteric background, are all covered here.

Available at bookstores and natural food stores nationwide or order your copy directly by sending cost of item plus $2.50 shipping/handling ($.75 s/h for each additional copy ordered at the same time) to:

Lotus Press, PO Box 325, Twin Lakes, WI 53181 USA
toll free order line: 800 824 6396 • office phone: 262 889 856 • office fax: 262 889 2461
email: lotuspress@lotuspress.com • web site: www.lotuspress.com

Lotus Press is the publisher of a wide range of books and software in the field of alternative health, including Ayurveda, Chinese medicine, herbology, aromatherapy, Reiki and energetic healing modalities. Request our free book catalog.

Herbs and other natural health products and information are often available at natural food stores or metaphysical bookstores. If you cannot find what you need locally, you can contact one of the following sources of supply.

Sources of Supply:

The following companies have an extensive selection of useful products and a long track-record of fulfillment. They have natural body care, aromatherapy, flower essences, crystals and tumbled stones, homeopathy, herbal products, vitamins and supplements, videos, books, audio tapes, candles, incense and bulk herbs, teas, massage tools and products and numerous alternative health items across a wide range of categories.

WHOLESALE:

Wholesale suppliers sell to stores and practitioners, not to individual consumers buying for their own personal use. Individual consumers should contact the RETAIL supplier listed below. Wholesale accounts should contact with business name, resale number or practitioner license in order to obtain a wholesale catalog and set up an account.

Lotus Light Enterprises, Inc.
PO Box 1008
Silver Lake, WI 53170 USA
262 889 8501 (phone)
262 889 8591 (fax)
800 548 3824 (toll free order line)
Website: www.lotuslight.com
email: lotuslight@lotuspress.com

RETAIL:

Retail suppliers provide products by mail order direct to consumers for their personal use. Stores or practitioners should contact the wholesale supplier listed above.

Internatural
PO Box 489
Twin Lakes, WI 53181 USA
800 643 4221 (toll free order line)
262 889 8581 office phone
EMAIL: internatural@internatural.com
WEBSITE: www.internatural.com

Website includes an extensive annotated catalog of more than 14,000 items that can be ordered "online" for your convenience 24 hours a day, 7 days a week.